magnet therapy illustrated

● ● ● ● ● ● ● ●

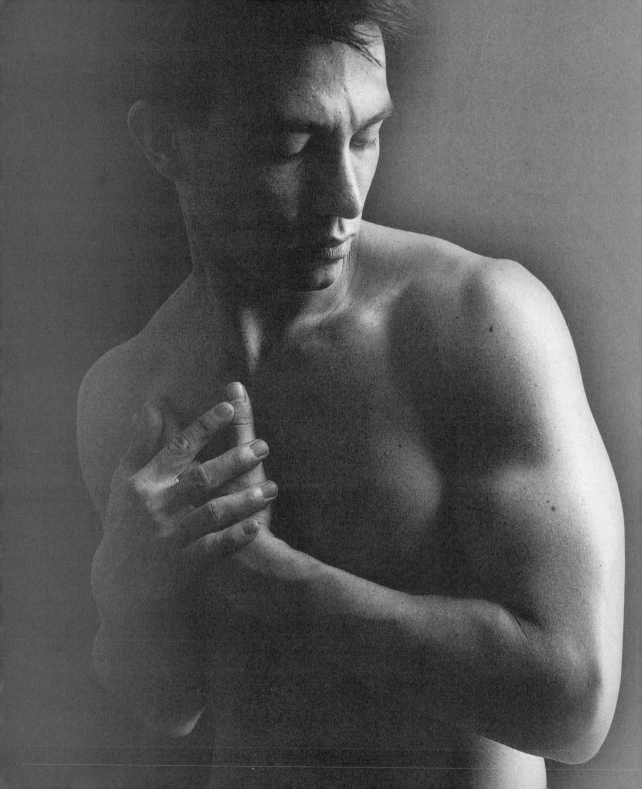

magnet therapy illustrated

● ● ● ● ● ● ● ● ● ● ● ●

Natural Healing and Pain Relief

Using Magnets

PETER ROSE

Photography by Laura Knox

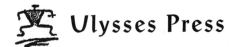 Ulysses Press

This book is dedicated to my partner, Joy, for her loyalty and support.
Also to the memory of those who have passed on before us. To my father
Bill Rose, my dear mother Olive Rose, my much-loved son Ben Rose and
to a man who was an inspiration to all who knew him, Simon Lyne.

Text copyright © Peter Rose 2001
Photographs copyright © Laura Knox 2001
This edition copyright © Eddison Sadd Editions 2001

The right of Peter Rose to be identified as the author of this
work has been asserted by him in accordance with the
Copyright, Designs and Patents Act 1988.

Published in the United States in 2001 by
Ulysses Press
P.O. Box 3440
Berkeley, CA 94703
www.ulyssespress.com

First published as *Magnet Healing* in the United Kingdom in
2001 by Time-Life Books

Library of Congress Card Number 00-110581
ISBN 1-56975-260-5
Printed in Canada

10 9 8 7 6 5 4 3 2 1

Cover photography: Lisette Le Bon/SuperStock (front) and
Laura Knox (back)
Cover design: Sarah Levin

Please Note
This book has been written and published strictly for
informational purposes, and in no way should be used as a
substitute for consultation with health care professionals. You
should not consider educational material herein to be the
practice of medicine or to replace consultation with a
physician or other medical practitioner. The author and
publisher are providing you with information in this work so
that you can have the knowledge and can choose, at your own
risk, to act on that knowledge. The author and publisher also
urge all readers to be aware of their health status and to
consult health care professionals before beginning any health
program, including changes in dietary habits.

Contents

Introduction

Magnet therapy is an established form of natural healing – like acupuncture and shiatsu – that is now beginning to gain wide acceptance in the western world. Its action can be described as slow-release "acupuncture" without the needles, using magnetism to provide a non-invasive and non-chemical treatment for the relief of pain and for the improvement of our general well-being, without causing additional pain.

The most commonly used healthcare magnets are small, disc magnets, available from pharmacies. They are known as permanent magnets, which means that they are still magnetic even though whatever it was that made them magnetic in the first place has been removed. They are usually supplied with a self-adhesive patch designed to hold the north-seeking pole against the skin. Placed on specific points on the skin and by working on the meridians, or channels of energy, the magnets balance out and improve the energy and blood flow in the body over a period of time. There are also many other types of self-help magnetic products available, such as magnetic bandages and shoe insoles (see pages 12–13).

In most simple cases, magnet therapy can be self-administered and it works extremely well in conjunction with other natural therapies, speeding up recovery time and alleviating pain. It is an inexpensive form of self-healing – the only cost is the magnets themselves – and for treating minor injuries and health problems no medical knowledge is required. All the information you need about the subject and where to position the magnets to treat a variety of common conditions is given in this book.

Relieving pain

The importance of pain relief should not be underestimated; it is not only worthwhile but necessary. Although it may be true that for some patients a change in lifestyle would eliminate certain pain, such change is only possible for those with enough self-esteem to acknowledge the need for it. But pain destroys self-esteem, which is why a good therapist seeks to relieve pain first, then moves on to investigate the condition fully and treat it accordingly.

A brief history of magnet therapy

Magnet therapy and the appreciation of the power of magnets have a long history. The magnetic properties of lodestones (naturally magnetic rocks) were recorded by the Greek philosopher Thales of Miletus in around 600 BCE, but magnets were known about long before they were mentioned in modern western writings. It has been suggested that ancient man had magnetically sensitive material in his nose, giving him a form of built-in compass. This could be the origin of the saying, "Best to just follow your nose!" So it may be true to say that the use of magnets is as old as humankind itself.

The ancient Chinese almost certainly used magnets and magnetic material to try to improve the flow of *chi* (also spelled *qi* or *ki*), the internal energy that flows around channels or meridians in the body, and some records claim that in the second century CE, Chinese sailors used magnets for navigation. The *Atharva-Veda*, the sacred ancient writings of Hinduism, refers to magnets being used to stop bleeding, while Cleopatra supposedly wore a small magnet on her forehead to preserve her fabled beauty.

Much later, in sixteenth-century Europe, Paracelsus, the Swiss alchemist and physician, wrote: "There are qualities in a magnet and one of these qualities is that the magnet also attracts all material humors that are in the human system. The magnet therefore is very useful in all inflammations, influxes and ulcerations in diseases of the bowels and uterus, in internal as well as external diseases." Around the same time, the physician Dr William Gilbert reputedly prescribed magnets for Queen Elizabeth I. Just over a century later in Switzerland, Dr Franz Mesmer conducted trials, experiments and treatments that used magnets for therapeutic benefits, and, in Britain, Dr Samuel Hahnemann, the founder of homeopathic medical practices, advocated the use of magnets for healing.

More recently, in 1862, Louis Pasteur discovered that the earth's magnetic field exercised a positive effect on the growth of plants. Today, electromagnetic devices, such as MRI scans (magnetic resonance imaging) and microwave therapy are commonplace in modern hospitals. So, although we appear to have come a long way since lodestones, magnetism still forms the basis of much advanced medical invention.

What is magnetism?

Magnetism is an energy, a force, that affects all of our lives all of the time. It has the ability to move things to which it is not connected physically. For example, the earth has a huge magnetic field, as have the sun and the moon. The seas' tides are caused by the magnetic influence of the moon and its interaction with the magnetic field of the earth. Recent research has shown that butterflies use an in-built magnetic compass to find their way during migration. Each year, Monarch butterflies fly 4,000 kilometers (2,500 miles) south from their breeding grounds in the US to spend the winter in Mexico. But if they were to be exposed to reversed magnetic fields, they would be unable to locate the right direction.

A horseshoe magnet showing the north and south poles and the energy flow between them.

The effects of magnetism

A magnet has the power to exert magnetic influence, which means that it has the power to cause an unattached object to move in relation to the magnet. That means it will either attract or repel other objects that it comes into contact with. The effect that magnetic forces have is to cause molecules to align themselves in a more orderly fashion than normal, rather like the difference between an unruly mob and guardsmen on parade. Every molecule has an alignment, or an order. These are usually different from those of neighboring molecules, but magnetic forces cause the molecules to line up in the same way relative to each other. In iron bars, for example, magnetic forces can cause the whole bar to become magnetic. By placing small magnets on the strategic acupuncture points of the body, we can use this power of alignment to help the body make a quicker recovery than it would do on its own and relieve physical pain caused by all sorts of problems (see pages 42–101).

Magnetic poles

The magnetic poles are the ends of a magnet, whether a rod, horseshoe or bar-shaped magnet, where the external magnetic field is the strongest. If a bar magnet is suspended in the earth's magnetic field, it will orientate itself in a north–south direction. The pole that seeks the north is called the north magnetic pole; the pole that seeks the south is called the south magnetic pole.

Like poles repel, so if you were to place a south pole close to another south pole, the magnets would try to push away from each other. Unlike poles attract, so if you were to place a north pole of one magnet close to the south pole of another magnet, the poles would be attracted and try to stick to each other. Energy flows from one end of a magnet to the other and all around it. If you were to cut a bar magnet into two, you would end up with two separate magnets, each with their own north and south poles.

Measuring magnets

Healthcare magnets come in a range of different strengths and are usually measured in gauss, but may also be measured in teslas per square metre (one tesla equals 10,000 gauss). The most useful for magnet therapy are between 500 and 15,000 gauss. An easy way to measure magnets is to compare the weights that different magnets can pick up.

The strength of the magnet required for magnet therapy depends on a number of factors, such as the severity of the injury. Magnets are very powerful healers, and strong magnets can even be used, by professional therapists, to assist the healing of broken bones.

The magnetic force exerted between the poles of two different magnets is said to follow "inverse square law," which means that if you double the distance between the poles of two different magnets, the force felt is reduced to a quarter. Applying this principle to magnet therapy, the further away the magnet is from the body, the smaller the magnetic force exerted on the site of pain. This means that, while 500 gauss magnets are useful for influencing the blood vessels that lie close to the surface of the skin, stronger magnets are needed for the healing processes deeper inside the body.

The inverse square law shows that as the distance between the magnet and its object is doubled (from A to B), its power is reduced by a quarter. This principle is also true when using magnets for healing.

Electricity and muscles

A close relationship exists between electricity and magnetism, and it is this relationship that is exploited in magnet therapy.

Electricity flowing along a wire produces a magnetic field around the wire. Also, if a magnet is rotated inside a coil of wire, electricity is generated in that wire. We need certain materials to make electrical generators, but the relationship between magnetic fields and electrical impulses is always present, whatever the materials. One of the very earliest experiments used to confirm the presence of electricity in muscles involved making the leg of a dead frog twitch when a small current of electricity was passed through the muscle.

Simply put, muscles are collections of tube-like fibers bound together in bundles. The fibers consist of thickly packed, long, thin contractile cells. Each fiber bundle is wrapped in a covering of tissue, called the perimysium. Each muscle is made up of several bundles of fibers separated from each other by yet another layer of tissue, called the deep fascia. Inside these bundles there are blood vessels and nerves. The brain sends signals to the muscles by causing an electrical impulse to travel along the nerves. To hold a muscle contracted requires forty nerve impulses per second – that is, 2,400 electrical impulses per minute.

Blood vessels bring in the chemicals needed for the muscles to do their work and carry away waste by-products, while the nerves are the electrical wiring circuitry, enabling that work to be done. Electricity in the body is generated by chemical interactions in specialist cells which send impulses racing down the nerves. Within every cell in the body there are molecules of fluid, which are generally random in their line-up (orientation) compared to each other, but magnetic forces can cause them to line up in order. Magnets affect the nerves (electrical "wiring") and the alignment of blood molecules within the blood vessels, improving the flow of electricity along these nerves and quickening the reaction time taken to get a muscle to move. Improved blood flow improves energy delivery and waste removal from a muscle (see also pages 35–39).

Healing magnets

There are several kinds of magnet that can be used for health purposes. The most common kinds are described on these pages, with recommendations for their use. Don't forget that magnets will also affect all electrical equipment, such as hearing implants. Magnets can also affect magnetic-strip data-storage devices, including credit cards, so be careful how you store and use them.

Warning
Never use magnets if you are dependent on a heart pacemaker.

Small spot magnets
The most commonly used healthcare magnets are small spot magnets of between 500 and 1,800 gauss. The range available from specialist outlets is far greater, but the most common and most useful is the 1,000 gauss. These magnets are usually supplied with a self-adhesive patch designed to hold the north-seeking pole against the skin.

These are of great use in situations where there is a need to improve local circulation. This can be for cramp, and bumps and bruises with no actual bleeding, internal or external. They are also useful for sprains and overstretched ligaments, for migraines and headaches. Research has indicated that many migraines involve a shortage of blood in certain areas of the brain, and so placement of small magnets as indicated on pages 42–101 will be beneficial in these cases. Small spot magnets are mostly used for acute conditions, but they can also be used for chronic cramp. Simply placing a magnet at the center of a painful area and then encircling it with more spot magnets will improve recovery rates.

Small spot magnets of around 1,000 gauss in strength are typically used for magnetic healing therapy.

Large magnets
Large magnets are used to try to influence the flow of energy through the whole body, but even large magnets have a limited power to send a magnetic field deep into the body. Extremely powerful magnetic fields are dangerous and so the use of these larger magnets

should be restricted to sessions supervised by qualifed practitioners. The smaller "spot" magnets are safe, unless you have a pacemaker or other electrically powered life-support mechanism, and are generally just as effective as the use of large single magnets.

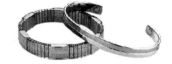

Magnetic bandages

Magnetic bandages and straps, and bandages or supports that contain magnets, are best used in cases of injury after all bleeding has stopped, to improve the flow of healing nutrients to the damaged area. They can also be used to strengthen areas of weakness, since repaired (scar) tissue is never quite as strong as the original material. It is helpful to give additional support to places that have suffered in the past, in particular, knees, wrists, elbows and shoulders.

Magnetic bandages specifically designed for certain parts of the body, such as this head bandage, are easy to use.

Other magnets

Head bandages that contain magnets can be used in conjunction with correctly placed spot magnets, for relief from head pain. Magnetic earrings, that are held in place by the attraction between two magnets placed either side of the earlobe, can also be used to gain specifically desired effects.

Magnetic wrist bracelets for travel sickness can be a great help, but it is important to keep the magnets located over the correct position (see pages 98–99). The bracelet should not be so loose that it can move around the wrist. For wrist sprains and strains use magnetic support bandages.

Shoe insoles used to apply magnetic energy to particular points on the soles of the feet work on the principles of reflexology. There are a range of these insoles available, and all have differing positions and strengths of magnets (see pages 109–110 for suppliers of magnetic products).

Mattresses or pillows containing magnets aid relaxation and blood flow while at rest, and are best used for general recovery and relief of chronic conditions.

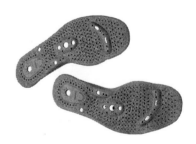

Magnetic bracelets are commonly used for travel sickness, as they put pressure on specific points.

Pressure exerted on reflexology points by magnets in shoe insoles can be used to treat certain conditions.

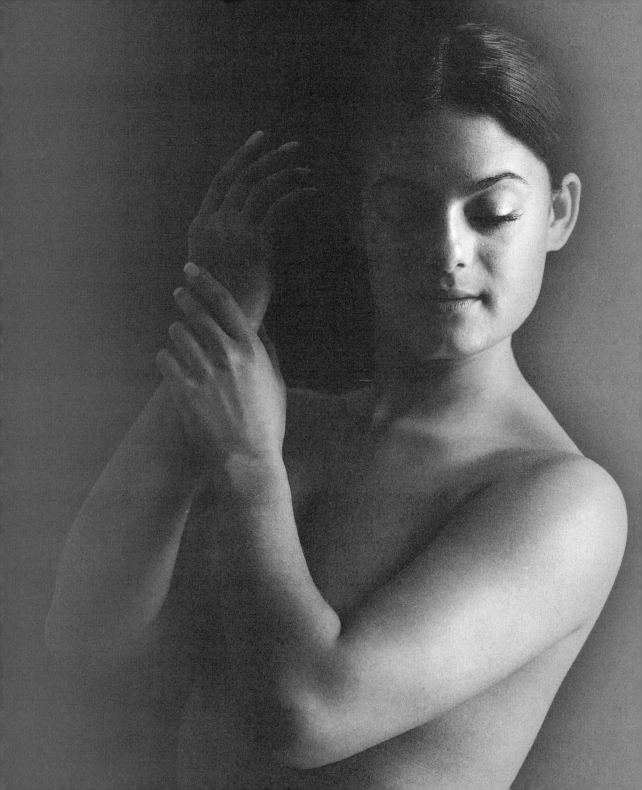

Part one **How magnet therapy works**

• • • • • • • • • • • • • • • •

This section of the book includes information on how to use magnets to speed recovery from injury and ill-health. There are two main ways in which magnets can be used for health: using them on acupuncture points as specific-point continuous treatment, in a similar way to shiatsu or reflexology treatments, or to improve the flow of blood.

By applying small magnets to particular points on the body, the meridians (energy pathways) can be unblocked and chi (life energy) can flow unrestricted. The meridians are channels which run all over the body. When they become blocked, chi cannot flow freely and illness results. By using the healing power of magnets on specific points along twelve of these meridians, a range of common conditions can be treated. The points indicated in this chapter are the same as those which are used in acupuncture treatments, and they are taken from the ancient system of traditional Chinese medicine.

The second way in which magnets can be used in this context is to improve the flow of blood. This is achieved by the ability of magnets to align molecules in blood cells so they can move more easily around the body. The following pages show you simple ways to use magnets to help relieve pain and discomfort caused by many common ailments.

• • • • • • • • • • • • • • • •

When to use magnets

Most of the treatments described in this book are done using small magnets. Placed on the body's acupuncture points they can help improve the flow of energy (see pages 22–34) and the blood flow around the body (see pages 35–39); using larger magnets influences the overall balance of energy within the body (see pages 41–42); and using "magnetized" water alters the flow of fluids, such as blood, internally (see page 106).

Preventative therapy

Magnet therapy can also be preventative. The repair tissue of old injuries is usually only sixty to seventy per cent as strong as the original tissue. So, if you strain a known weak point, apply magnets around the site of the injury as soon as possible after its recurrence to prevent further pain and problems in the future.

Healing scars

Magnets may be placed over scars, provided the skin is well healed and has not bled for at least seven days. Although magnets should not be used on partially healed wounds, such as scabs, they can be applied to scar tissue where the skin has rejoined and the wound completely healed. There have been reports that using magnets over scar tissue improves the regeneration of "normal" skin to lessen the visible scar.

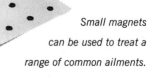

Small magnets can be used to treat a range of common ailments.

16

Contraindications

Always consult your medical practitioner in cases of severe or persistent health problems, and especially in cases of acute (sudden) pain or problems that persist for more than a few days, before using magnet therapy. Never use magnets with pacemakers or other electromechanical implants in the body. Be aware that powerful magnets can affect all electromagnetic devices, such as battery-operated clocks and watches. If the magnets are very powerful, even the magnetized strips on credit cards can be affected.

More specifically, do not use the stick-on types of magnet on broken skin or skin rashes. Some people do have an intolerance to the adhesives used on certain sticking plasters, or even to the type of coating on the magnets themselves. If the skin becomes irritated or inflamed, remove the magnets and wash the affected area with warm, soapy water. The problem should clear up quickly, but if it persists for more than three days, consult your medical practitioner.

Avoiding embarrassment

In treatments where the magnets are visible and may cause embarrassment, such as on the face, remove the magnets during the day but leave any hidden ones in place. Replace the visible magnets at night and when you are alone.

If the adhesive tape leaves a mark on the skin after removal, this can be washed off with soap and water or make-up remover. If the area around a magnet becomes inflamed or itchy, remove the magnet. Do not apply magnets to areas of inflamed, itchy or broken skin.

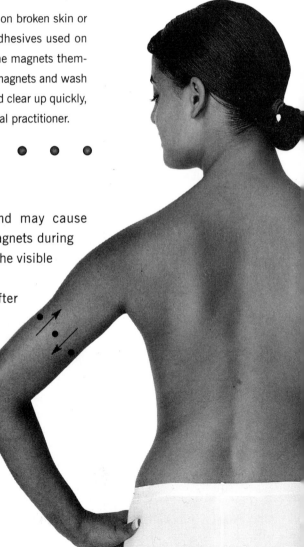

Placing a ring of magnets around a limb between the injury and the heart is believed to improve blood flow and energy flow around the body. This illustration shows blood flowing away from and towards the heart.

The meridians

The meridians are the channels, or pathways, of energy that circulate round the body. Although the maps of these meridians do not show how they are connected, the ancient Chinese who first drew them understood that they do link to each other in an orderly fashion, creating a continuous flow around the body. Interruptions to the smooth flow of this energy are associated with ill-health, indicated by pain, stiffness or swelling. Shiatsu, reflexology, acupuncture and many other well-known health-improvement therapies all utilize the principle of meridians.

In standard acupuncture theory, there are twelve major meridians and an extra eight channels and fifteen "collaterals." In magnet therapy, we are only concerned with the so-called "classical" meridians: twelve major channels (lung, large intestine, stomach, spleen, heart, small intestine, bladder, kidney, pericardium, triple heater, gall bladder and liver), and two extra pathways (governing vessel and conception vessel).

Although meridian pathways are often depicted on one side of the body for simplicity, they all run symmetrically on both sides of the body. When using magnets for healing, you may, therefore, use them on the relevant points on both sides.

How energy flows through the meridians

Lung meridian to large intestine to stomach to spleen to heart to small intestine to bladder to kidney to pericardium to triple heater to gall bladder to liver and back to lung.

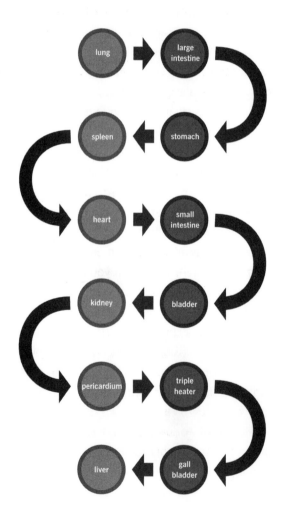

Each meridian is named after an organ or function connected to its energy flow. While most people are familiar with the standard organs of the body, some explanation of pericardium, triple heater, governing vessel and conception vessel may help.

Pericardium

In the human body, the pericardium is the membrane surrounding the heart. It contains a small amount of fluid and prevents friction between the heart and the lungs and ribs when the heart beats, hence its alternative names of "heart constrictor" and "heart governor" meridian. It runs down the inside of the arm and is worked on in the treatment of cardiac problems, palpitations, restlessness and mental disturbance.

Triple heater

Also referred to as the "triple warmer," the triple heater is a function of the body's energy system rather than a physical organ, producing and delivering heat energy to all parts of the body. It is divided into three sections: the upper burner (the area of the meridian covering the chest, heart and lungs), the middle burner (the area between the diaphragm and navel) and the lower burner (below the navel). It is used in the treatment of abdominal distention, edema, deafness, tinnitus and congestion.

Conception vessel

The conception vessel runs up the center line of the body. Like the governing vessel, this meridian starts in the lower abdomen, where it is inaccessible. It runs down to the anus and then becomes accessible as it runs up the front of the body. Since it passes directly through the reproductive organs, its name is easily understood.

Governing vessel

Like the triple heater, this is a function of the body's energy system rather than a physical organ. The meridian runs up the center line of the back of the body over the top of the head and meets the conception vessel, when the tongue is pressed to the roof of the mouth. The deep, inaccessible parts of the meridian are at its beginning and end. The connection between the brain and the lower abdomen, which is both the body's center of gravity and its most important part in energy terms, is the reason this meridian is called the governing vessel. It is, however, of limited use in magnet therapy.

These illustrations show how the major meridians and the two further pathways – the conception vessel and the governor vessel – are situated in the body. These are shown in further detail on pages 24–32.

Energy flows around the whole body, passing from one meridian to another, to complete a circuit. Remember that although practitioners may, for example, speak of "liver" energy, this is some of the available energy flowing in the liver meridian at a particular time. It is not energy unique to the liver, but is part of a whole circuit. The routes of the meridians and the positions of the points are the same on both the left and right side of the body. Only one side of each is shown here for the sake of simplicity.

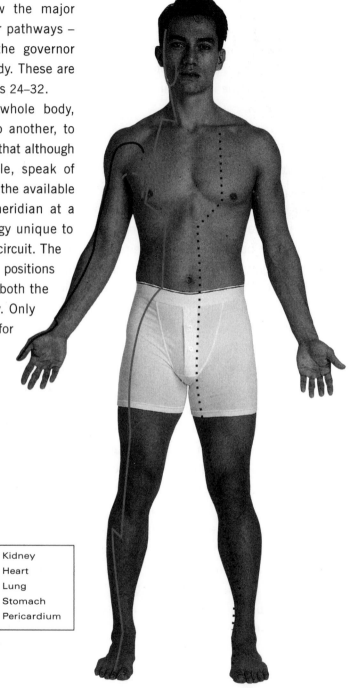

......	Kidney
....	Heart
▬▬	Lung
▬▬	Stomach
▬ ▬	Pericardium

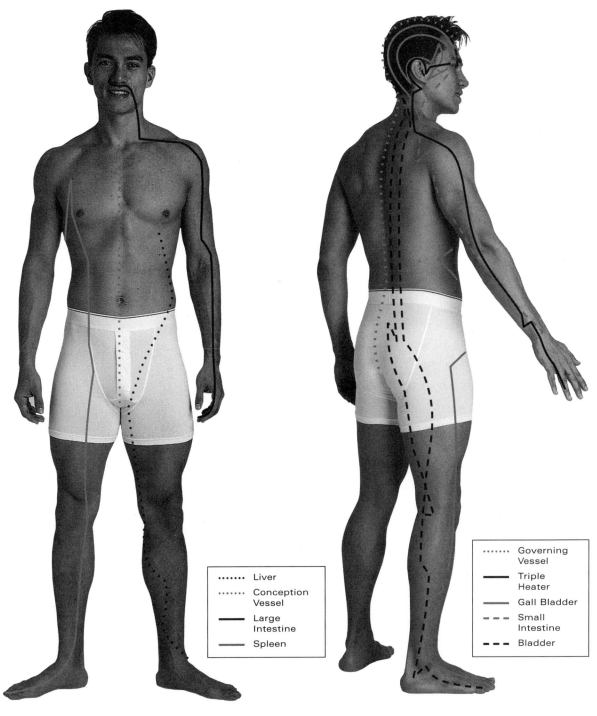

·······	Liver
·······	Conception Vessel
——	Large Intestine
——	Spleen

·······	Governing Vessel
——	Triple Heater
——	Gall Bladder
– – –	Small Intestine
– – –	Bladder

Energy flow

The ancient Chinese believed that our chi, or energy, was made up of three parts. The first is the energy we are born with. The second part is the energy we inherit from our parents and which is supplemented by the love we receive from those around us – this energy grows during our lives as it is fed by positive emotions, by love and nurturing, but it is also reduced by negative emotions, by pain and negative life experiences. The third and final part is the energy we get from food and from the air we breathe – this energy is environmental, extracted from the physical world around us.

If you consider this breakdown of energy from a different angle, the first type is the minimum needed to sustain the automatic processes of physical life, the second allows us to have emotions, and the third enables us to be active in a physical world. Modern conventional medicine practices on the third type of energy, while prayer and faith-healing are believed to work on a combination of the first and second. Magnet therapy, like acupuncture, works on a combination of the second and third.

Points on the meridian pathways

There are points along the meridians where it is possible to speed up or slow down the flow of energy within the meridians. Often applying external energy will allow a point to regain its balance. Shiatsu requires the application of pressure to a point, allowing the system to use that energy to balance itself according to its needs. Acupuncture uses needles instead of pressure. Generally, if it is possible to determine the condition of energy flowing, then sluggish flow needs stimulation and tonification, while excessive flow needs sedation. Many of the treatments that utilize these energy flows work on the same principle, that if the flow of energy is harmonized, the body will restore its own balance and well-being. The key word is *balance*: if the flow is correct, then the harmonization of the various interrelated functions of the organs of the body will also be correct.

How magnets affect energy flow

Ill-health, in terms of energy in the meridians, is seen to be due to the stagnation of energy in one part of the system and its depletion in another. Which is cause and which is effect does not really matter when it comes to improving and balancing the flow of energy.

Healing magnets work like slow-release acupuncture needles. By placing them on specific points along the meridians you will allow their energy to induce a harmony of energy flow in the body that is essential to good health. They are also specifically designed so that you can attach them to acupuncture points all over the body.

Although a skilled acupuncturist will work on certain meridians only when they are most active, this may not be the case with practitioners of other more generalized disciplines, like magnet therapy. In specific-point magnet therapy, where the magnets are applied to particular areas of the body, the magnets are usually left in place for no less than twenty-four hours, so all the time periods for all the meridians (see right) are covered. Magnets used on specific areas provide a continuous release of energy over a relatively long time, which can be anything from twenty-four hours to ten days, balancing and harmonizing the flow of energy gently and evenly. This then dispels the stagnation and depletion of energy.

The flow of energy around the meridians is continuous, but there are certain times when it is more active than others. Equally, it can be sluggish when we are ill. Magnet therapy improves that flow.

Energy timetable

There is a time period each day when a large proportion of the body's energy is in a specific meridian. The body adjusts its energy flow according to the time zone it is in, so the times given below are relevant wherever you are. Jet lag occurs when the body clock is adjusting to time-zone changes.

MERIDIAN	TIME
lung	3 am to 5 am
large intestine	5 am to 7 am
stomach	7 am to 9 am
spleen	9 am to 11 am
heart	11 am to 1 pm
small intestine	1 pm to 3 pm
bladder	3 pm to 5 pm
kidney	5 pm to 7 pm
pericardium	7 pm to 9 pm
triple heater	9 pm to 11 pm
gall bladder	11 pm to 1 am
liver	1 am to 3 am

Meridian points used in magnet therapy

Conception vessel

The key points on the conception vessel meridian,
and the conditions they may be used to treat.

CV 4 general tonic for
the energy system;
irregular menstruation
CV 5 irregular
menstruation;
abdominal distention
CV 6 abdominal
distention with pain;
irregular menstruation
CV 8 abdominal pain
(it may be difficult to
get a magnet to stick
to this point)
CV 12 vomiting;
abdominal distention
CV 13 vomiting;
abdominal distention
CV 16 asthma; coughs;
vomiting
CV 17 bronchial
asthma
CV 21 coughs; asthma;
pain and swelling in
throat
CV 24 toothache

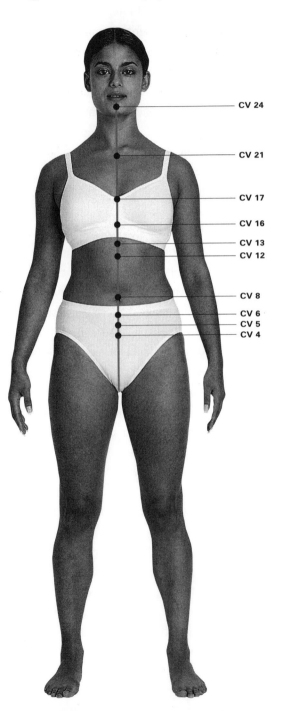

CV 24

CV 21

CV 17

CV 16

CV 13
CV 12

CV 8

CV 6
CV 5
CV 4

Governing vessel

The key points on the governing vessel meridian, and the conditions they may be used to treat. Other points could also be beneficial, but it is not possible to adhere magnets to hair or to lightly mobile areas of the face.

GV 3 lumbago

GV 4 lumbago; abdominal swelling

GV 5 back pain in general; lumbago in particular

GV 8 general back pain

GV 9 chest and back pain; general stiffness in spine

GV 11 coughs; stiff back; anxiety

GV 13 headache; stiff back

GV 14 heatstroke; fever; asthma

GV 14
GV 13
GV 11
GV 9
GV 8
GV 5
GV 4
GV 3

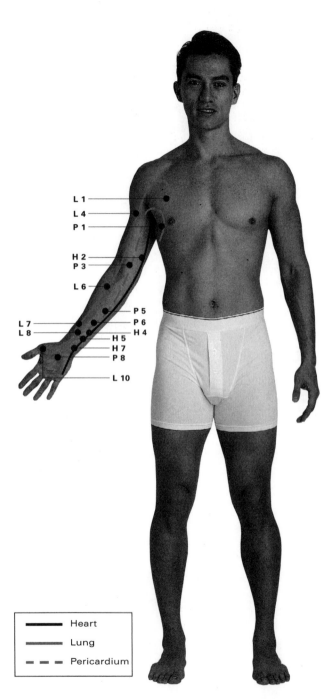

L 1
L 4
P 1
H 2
P 3
L 6
P 5
L 7   P 6
L 8   H 4
       H 5
       H 7
       P 8
L 10

Heart
Lung
Pericardium

Pericardium

The key points on the pericardium meridian, and the conditions they may be used to treat. Place magnets on these points on both sides of the body.

P 1 breast problems; sensation of suffocation in chest
P 3 pain in elbow and arms; tremors in hands and arms
P 5 vomiting; pain and cramp in arms, wrists and hands

P 6 vomiting; nausea; travel sickness; morning sickness
P 8 cardiac pain; fungal infection in hands and feet

Lung

The key points on the lung meridian, and the conditions they may be used to treat. Place magnets on these points on both sides of the body.

L 1 pain in chest, shoulder and upper back
L 4 coughs; shortness of breath; pain in chest
L 6 coughs; asthma; swelling in elbows and arms

L 7 headaches; stiff neck; asthma
L 8 pain in chest; sore throat; pain in wrists and hands
L 10 coughs; asthma; sore throat

Heart

The key points on the heart meridian, and the conditions they may be used to treat. Place magnets on these points on both sides of the body.

H 2 pain in shoulders and arms
H 4 pain in chest; sudden hoarseness in voice

H 5 dizziness; blurred vision; sore throat; pain in wrists and arms
H 7 pain in chest; irritability

Small intestine

The key points on the small intestine meridian, and the conditions they may be used to treat. Place magnets on these points on both sides of the body.

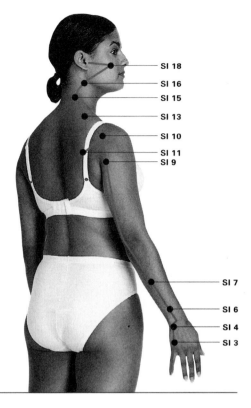

SI 3 headaches; stiff neck

SI 4 headaches; stiff neck

SI 6 shoulder ache; blurred vision; combined pain in back, arms and elbows

SI 7 pain in fingers; pain in neck

SI 9 pain in shoulder blade; difficulty in shoulder and arm movement

SI 10 pain and weakness in shoulder and arms

SI 11 pain in shoulder blade, elbows and arms

SI 13 stiffness in shoulder blade

SI 15 coughs; asthma

SI 16 sore throat; stiff neck

SI 18 toothache

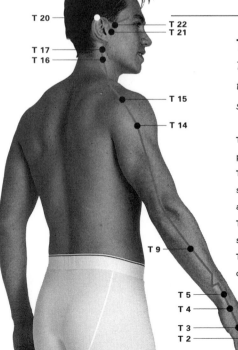

Triple heater

The key points on the triple heater meridian, and the conditions they may be used to treat. Place magnets on these points on both sides of the body.

T 2 headaches; sore throat; pain in hands and arms

T 3 headaches; tinnitus; sore throat; pain in elbows and arms

T 4 pain in wrist; pain in shoulders and arms

T 5 headaches; pain in cheeks; tinnitus; loss of movement in elbows and arms

T 9 toothache

T 14 pain in arms

T 15 pain in shoulders and arms; stiffness in neck

T 16 dizziness; blurred vision

T 17 tinnitus; swelling in cheeks

T 20 redness and pain in eyes; toothache

T 21 tinnitus; toothache

T 22 tinnitus; headaches

27

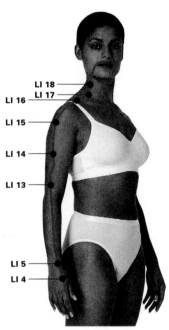

LI 18
LI 17
LI 16
LI 15
LI 14
LI 13
LI 5
LI 4

Large intestine

The key points on the large intestine meridian, and the conditions they may be used to treat. Place magnets on these points on both sides of the body.

LI 4 most upper body pains; migraine; headaches; toothache

LI 5 headaches; toothache; pain in wrists and hands

LI 13 pain in elbows and arms

LI 14 pain and loss of movement in elbows and arms

LI 15 pain in elbows and arms; problems in shoulders

LI 16 pain in shoulders

LI 17 sore throat

LI 18 coughs; sore throat

Kidney

The key points on the kidney meridian, and the conditions they may be used to treat. Place magnets on these points on both sides of the body.

K 1 dizziness; blurred vision; headaches

K 2 pain and swelling in feet; cystitis; sore throat

K 3 cystitis; toothache; sore throat

K 7 pain and stiffness in lower back; abdominal distention

K 9 pain in legs; spasm in leg muscles

K 10 pain in thigh

muscles; pain in knees

K 16 vomiting; abdominal distension; abdominal pain

K 17 constipation; diarrhea

K 19 abdominal pain

K 21 abdominal pain; vomiting

K 27 chest pain; coughs; asthma; breathing and lung problems in general

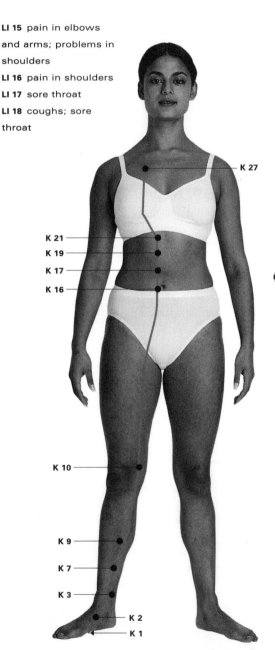

K 27

K 21
K 19
K 17
K 16

K 10

K 9

K 7

K 3

K 2
K 1

Spleen

The key points on the spleen meridian, and the conditions they may be used to treat. Place magnets on these points on both sides of the body.

Sp 3 gastric pain; feeling of sluggishness
Sp 6 general point for many problems, particularly digestive and menstrual pain
Sp 10 irregular menstruation
Sp 12 abdominal pain
Sp 14 pain near umbilicus
Sp 16 indigestion

Stomach

The key points on the stomach meridian, and the conditions they may be used to treat. Place magnets on these points on both sides of the body.

St 5 toothache
St 7 toothache
St 9 asthma; sore throat
St 10 asthma; sore throat
St 13 asthma; chest and back pain
St 16 coughs; asthma
St 26 abdominal pain; menstrual pain
St 27 cystitis; abdominal pain
St 28 cystitis
St 29 menstrual pain
St 32 pain and loss of mobility in legs
St 33 leg ache; loss of movement in knees
St 34 pain in and around knees
St 35 pain in knees
St 36 digestive problems in general
St 39 abdominal pain
St 40 chest pain; dizziness
St 41 pain in ankle joints
St 42 toothache; pain in feet
St 43 pain and swelling in feet
St 44 headaches; toothache

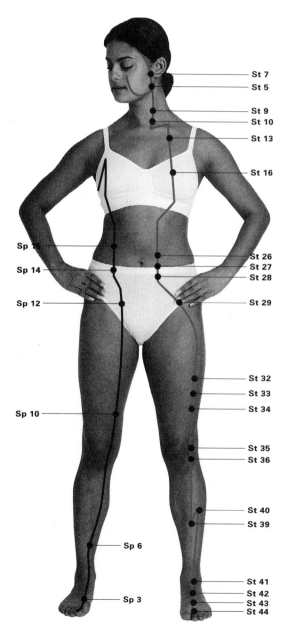

St 7
St 5
St 9
St 10
St 13
St 16
St 26
St 27
St 28
St 29
St 32
St 33
St 34
St 35
St 36
St 40
St 39
St 41
St 42
St 43
St 44

Sp 16
Sp 14
Sp 12
Sp 10
Sp 6
Sp 3

— Spleen
••••• Stomach

29

Bladder

The key points on the bladder meridian, and the conditions they may be used to treat. Place magnets on these points on both sides of the body.

B 10 stiff pain in neck or back of head
B 11 coughs; headaches; stiff neck
B 12 common cold; fever; headaches; neckache; backache
B 13 coughs; asthma; night sweats
B 14 full feeling in chest; headaches
B 15 panic; irritability; palpitations
B 16 abdominal pain
B 17 asthma; coughs; difficulty in breathing
B 18 blurred vision; disturbed sleep; back pain
B 19 back pain; chest pain
B 20 abdominal distention; indigestion

B 21 chest pain; indigestion
B 22 lumbago; irregular menstruation
B 23 backache; weak knees; blurred vision
B 26 lumbago
B 31 lumbago; sciatica
B 32 lumbago; sciatica; rheumatic pain in legs
B 33 rheumatic pain in legs; lumbago; sciatica
B 40 lower back pain; restricted hip movement
B 41 pain in shoulders, back and neck
B 43 coughs; asthma; indigestion
B 49 constipation
B 58 headaches; blurred vision; weakness in legs
B 62 headaches; dizziness; vertigo
B 65 headaches; rigid neck; blurred vision; dizziness

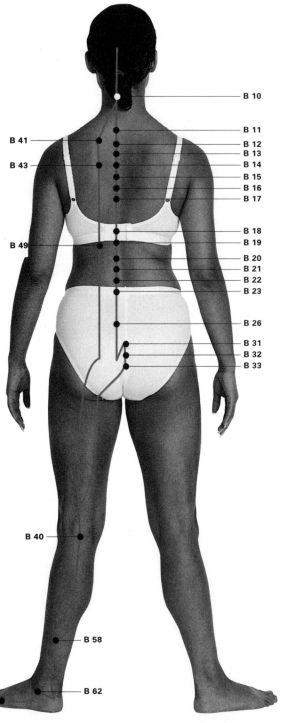

Gall bladder

The key points on the gall bladder meridian, and the conditions they may be used to treat. Place magnets on these points on both sides of the body.

GB 1 headaches; eye problems

GB 2 tinnitus; toothache; arthritis in jaw

GB 3 headaches; toothache; tinnitus

GB 10 headaches; toothache; tonsillitis

GB 11 headaches; earache; pain in neck; tinnitus

GB 12 toothache; facial stiffness

GB 20 headaches; dizziness; common cold; neck pain; stiff neck

GB 21 pain in shoulders and back; stiff neck

GB 25 pain in lower back

GB 26 pain in lower back; cystitis

GB 29 pain in back; hip problems

GB 30 sciatica; problems with hips; pain in lower back and hips

GB 31 pain in legs; problems with hormone and digestive enzyme production

GB 33 pain in knees; swelling in knees

GB 37 pain in legs and knees; eye disease

GB 40 pain in neck and chest; pain in ankles

GB 41 blurred vision; pain in chest; pain and swelling in feet

GB 42 pain in breast and chest; pain in eyes

GB 43 dizziness; chest pain; facial pain

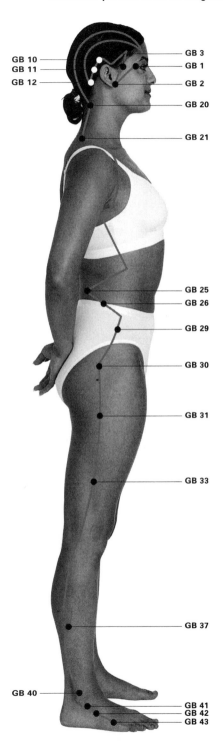

31

Liver

The key points on the liver meridian, and the conditions they may be used to treat. Place magnets on these points on both sides of the body.

Liv 2 eye problems; headaches; blurred vision; insomnia

Liv 3 headaches; vertigo

Liv 5 irregular menstruation; pain in legs; general skin problems

Liv 7 pain in knees

Liv 8 pain in lower abdomen; pain in thighs

Liv 9 irregular menstruation; pain in lower back with "referral" effect to lower abdomen

Liv 11 pain in legs and thighs

Liv 13 (on the side of the trunk halfway between the nipple and the umbilicus) indigestion; general tiredness; weakness of whole physical system

Liv 14 pain in chest

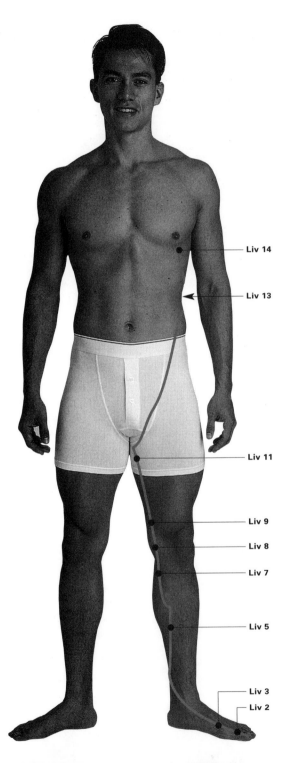

Liv 14

Liv 13

Liv 11

Liv 9

Liv 8

Liv 7

Liv 5

Liv 3

Liv 2

Using magnets on specific points

Magnets need to be placed with the north-seeking pole as close to the relevant acupuncture point as possible (see pages 24–32), although a precise location is not absolutely necessary to gain effective treatment. This is because the energy emanating from the magnets does so in all directions and so reaches out to the part of the meridian that will absorb it.

Locating acupuncture points

To treat a specific condition with magnets placed over acupuncture points, refer to pages 24–32, or check on the case examples that follow in Part Two to establish which points you are going to use. An easy way of locating a precise point is to press gently around the area where you expect it to be found with the end of a matchstick. Where the pressure causes the greatest pain is where you should place the magnet. Stick your magnets in place, north pole against the skin, and leave them there for five to seven days, or twenty-four hours after the pain has left you, whichever is the shorter. If a magnet comes off, when washing, for example, replace it using a new strip of medical adhesive tape to hold it in place. A thin surgical tape, such as Micropore, is good for this.

Selecting acupuncture points

If the problem you wish to treat has a number of different possible treatment points, such as abdominal distention or back pain, select eight points for your first wave of treatment, leave the magnets in place for five days, then move all or some of them to the other prescribed locations.

If a condition is chronic (long-term), rather than acute (sudden and severe), you will need to repeat the treatment several times, depending on the type of problem being treated and its severity. Each application should be left in place for five to seven days, with an interval of two days between each application.

Finding the north-seeking pole

There is sometimes confusion over which side of a therapy magnet to place against the skin because of the various ways in which manufacturers "label" the poles of their magnets. A skilled acupuncturist or shiatsu practitioner is able to evaluate the energy condition of the magnets without labeling, and knows which is the north-seeking pole to place against the skin, to stimulate, and which is the south-seeking pole, to sedate.

For home use, the simplest way to be sure that you are positioning the magnets correctly is to go by the manufacturer's labeling. Since most small magnets are supplied with the adhesive tape against the south-seeking pole, the north-seeking pole automatically faces the body. Some suppliers label the north-seeking pole red, and the south-seeking pole blue.

If the magnet becomes separated from its adhesive tape, take a second magnet with marked poles and place it close to the side of the magnet that is to be placed next to the skin. The north-seeking pole of the therapy magnet will be attracted to the south-seeking pole of the marked magnet and repelled by the north-seeking pole.

By holding the north-seeking pole of one magnet next to another, the north and south poles can be identified. The north-seeking pole of one will attract the south pole (top) and repel the north pole (bottom) of the other.

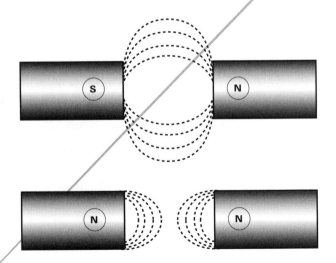

Blood flow

Blood is vital to life, and the efficiency with which our blood flows around the body has a huge effect on our health and well-being. There are normally about five to six liters of blood circulating around the body, and it is estimated that a red blood cell, which has a life span of approximately four months, is constantly traveling at an average speed of half a kilometer per hour. No wonder we have an expression about people having "tired blood"!

The role of blood

Our blood is, in effect, the transport system for the body, carrying essential goods to where they are needed and taking away waste products. If blood circulation is sluggish, delivery of those essential goods is sluggish and the stagnation of unwanted waste products can occur, which manifests itself in our bodies in a number of ways and may cause ill-health.

Blood flows around the body in tubes called blood vessels. There are two main kinds of blood vessels, which are arteries and veins. The arteries, the delivery system, carry blood away from the heart, while the veins, the waste collection system, transport blood back to the heart. The blood vessels become smaller as they divide up to reach the various parts of the body. At their smallest they are called capillaries, and these small tubes transfer the essential goods and waste products from and to the blood. The wall of a capillary is only one cell thick, so that oxygen and nutrients can cross this wall from the blood and into the body's cells. Carbon dioxide and other waste products cross back in the other direction, so the blood can carry them away for processing in the lungs, liver and kidneys.

Iron is an element that forms a key part of hemoglobin in red blood cells. It enables oxygen to be held in the blood and thus transported to where it is needed, mostly to the muscles and brain. Hemoglobin is red, giving blood its color. Other blood cells are white, and they fight disease.

The heart

The blood circulation system is driven by the heart, which is a pump capable of forcing blood through the entire body and along the smallest capillaries. If the heart becomes less efficient or the blood vessels become clogged or less flexible, the blood transport system becomes less efficient at delivering the nutrients and chemicals we use to drive our brain, heart and muscles. Healthy blood flow is vital to our survival: diseases of the heart and blood circulatory system are among the biggest health problems we face. And they are the cause of much pain, worry and discomfort.

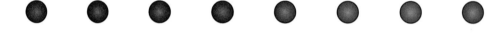

How magnets affect blood flow

Water makes up between sixty and seventy per cent of the human body, and the ability of magnetic fields to influence the flow of water can be seen all around us, from the ebb and flow of the tides to the use of electromagnetic induction coils to soften water. It stands to reason that magnets will directly affect our bodies, too.

Magnetic fields

Magnetic fields interact with the structure of human body cells to cause changes to the processing of proteins, hormones and enzymes. The changes are caused by the effect the magnetic field has on the outer wall of a cell, which is a double layer of molecules with complex molecules sandwiched in this double layer. Some of these complex molecules serve as channels to facilitate the transfer of oxygen and nutrients across cell walls. Although this all takes place at the molecular level, each minuscule change contributes to the overall effect.

Electromagnetic induction

Magnetic influence in the human body also creates electromagnetic induction within the cells, which improves the transfer of oxygen and nutrients across the cells. Electromagnetic induction is the process by which electricity is produced when a magnet is moved within a coil of wire, generating a small electric current. The energy from the magnetic field causes the electrons within the cell to vibrate; this is electricity. One of the basic laws of physics is that energy cannot be created or destroyed, only transformed. A magnet does not lose its power, however much electrical energy is generated in another material. In fact, electricity is generated only when the magnet moves relative to the coil of wire, and in order for the magnet to move, there must be a supply of energy to create the movement. It is this movement energy that is being transformed, leaving the actual magnet unchanged. How magnets create minute electrical currents in the cells of the human body cells is more complex; the cell itself provides the movement energy that is transformed into a tiny electrical charge.

Additional benefits of magnet therapy

There is some speculation that as well as aligning molecules in the blood and producing minute electrical currents in the body's cells, a magnetic field improves the ionic exchange of a cell, which allows waste products to leave a cell more efficiently. An ion is an electrically charged molecule. There are also people who believe that magnets affect the chemical (pH) balance within the body which, in turn, affects the chemical changes and composition of cell structures. However, this has not been proved by scientific research yet. Much more research remains to be done to determine why magnets have the beneficial effects that they do.

Improving blood flow

Placing a series of magnets around a tube that carries a semi-viscous fluid improves the flow of that fluid. Therefore, if magnets are placed 5 cm (2 in) apart around an arm, the flow of blood within the arm is improved. The level of improvement is dependent on a combination of many factors, including the strength of the magnets, the thickness of the arm, the layer of fat between the magnets and the blood vessels, the viscosity of the blood, and the combination of blood pressure and blood flow.

If magnets are placed on the body so that they, in effect, surround a part of a blood vessel on all sides, there will be an improvement in the blood flow at that point as the molecules of the blood realign themselves (see page 17). Hence they are of great benefit in conditions such as cramp and stiffness, where poor blood flow is the cause of discomfort.

Where to place the magnets

Where you position magnets depends on the nature of the problem. This is explained in more detail later, but a basic principle to follow is to place small magnets in a circle around the area where an improvement is desirable. If, for example, the problem is cramp in the lower arm, encircle the affected limb with magnets about 5 cm (2 in) apart and above the problem area, that is, between the heart and the problem area (see right). For pain in the back, place the magnets in a circle around the painful area, as shown right, to improve the blood flow in the capillaries. This will speed up the transport of nutrients to the injured site and the removal of waste products from it.

Theory and research

A great deal of research still needs to be done on the effects of magnetic fields on blood flow, as well as on the many aspects of the relationship between human beings and

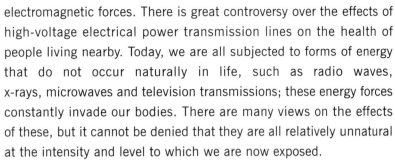

Placing magnets around the area of injury, such as on the back as shown here, or between the injury and the heart will improve blood flow and help the injury to heal.

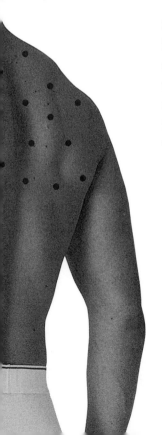

electromagnetic forces. There is great controversy over the effects of high-voltage electrical power transmission lines on the health of people living nearby. Today, we are all subjected to forms of energy that do not occur naturally in life, such as radio waves, x-rays, microwaves and television transmissions; these energy forces constantly invade our bodies. There are many views on the effects of these, but it cannot be denied that they are all relatively unnatural at the intensity and level to which we are now exposed.

The use of fixed magnets may restore some balance and normality in the body. It is possible that magnets used in the ways described in this book will help the body to cope with the increased numbers of free radicals that our bodies are faced with today. Free radicals are oxygen molecules missing an electron, which are unstable and seek to disrupt other molecules in the body. There is scope for further research into this area, but it has yet to be carried out.

Studies seem to indicate that the use of magnets may improve the quality of blood as well as its flow. This would mean even further benefits in using magnet therapy. Further beneficial effects may come from the normalization of localized abnormal electromagnetic forces. Since geopathic stress neutralizers seem to do this for a room, why should small fixed magnets not do the same on a very local level? However it works, there is much anecdotal evidence for the effectiveness of magnetic products including bandages, magnetic insoles in shoes, magnetic wrist bands and magnetic mattresses.

Warning

Do not use magnets where any bleeding – internal or external – is taking place (except for menstruation). Severed capillaries and blood vessels need a reduced blood flow and restricted local blood pressure in order to heal. Magnets will produce the opposite effect.

Large magnets

Research in India has shown that large magnets – those capable of lifting over 10 kg (22 lb) of magnetic material – affect the blood in a number of ways. Tests revealed that the iron content of the blood became active and a very weak electrical current was generated when a large magnet was placed in contact with the body. The process of electrically charging molecules (ionization) was increased, reducing clotting and increasing the rate of blood flow. Additional research has shown that large magnets improve the general quality of blood by speeding up the movement of hemoglobin in the red blood cells and reducing harmful deposits of both calcium and cholesterol in the blood vessels. There are also reports of increased hormonal activity and glandular activity; this is the reason for short periods of treatment in weak patients as increased hormonal activity would overload a weak metabolism.

It has also been claimed that large magnets can improve the functioning of the autonomic nervous system, which controls the involuntary actions of muscles. If this is the case, the function of the internal organs could be improved as a consequence, suggesting that larger magnets could be used in the treatment of more organic conditions, such as weakness of the liver or kidneys. However, treatment of this kind should only be carried out under professional guidance.

Treatment with large magnets

Large magnets are used in pairs so that, for example, one is held in the left hand with the south pole against the palm and the other in the right hand with the north pole against the palm.

The magnets are placed, for relatively short times, in specific positions on the body depending on the effect desired. The length of time will vary according to the severity of the condition being treated and the relative strength of the patient. For children, large magnets should be applied for no longer than five minutes at a time. As a general rule of thumb, the weaker the overall strength of the patient, the shorter the length of time that magnets should be used in a treatment session. Normally, treatment with large magnets should not exceed ten minutes per day. In extreme cases, treatment for chronic conditions should start with a session of five minutes per day and build up to twenty minutes twice a day until the desired effect is obtained.

Warning

- The use of large magnets is not recommended without seeking the advice of a trained magnet healer.
- Treatment with large magnets should not take place during pregnancy.
- Large magnets should not be used less than two hours after eating.

Handling and storage

Large magnets should be kept away from sensitive electronic equipment, and people fitted with pacemakers should not go near them. Modern materials used to manufacture large magnets are extremely strong magnetically but somewhat weak mechanically, so their handling is best left to those who have been specially trained. It is not advisable to attempt to treat yourself with large magnets.

Large magnets in such devices as loud speakers should not be removed for therapeutic purposes, as the materials used to make them and the strength of such magnets are unknown.

Treatment with large magnets

Large magnets are particularly useful for treating ailments of the nervous system, such as neuralgia and neuritis. The former, which is pain in the nerves, can affect most parts of the body and sometimes cause numbness. The latter is the inflammation of the nerves, also causing severe pain. The treatment for both conditions is the same, with the north-seeking pole of a magnet being applied at one end of the site of pain and the south-seeking pole of another magnet being applied at the other end. The strength and effect of large magnets, however, has not been fully researched, and it would be advisable to seek a trained magnet therapist before embarking on this form of treatment.

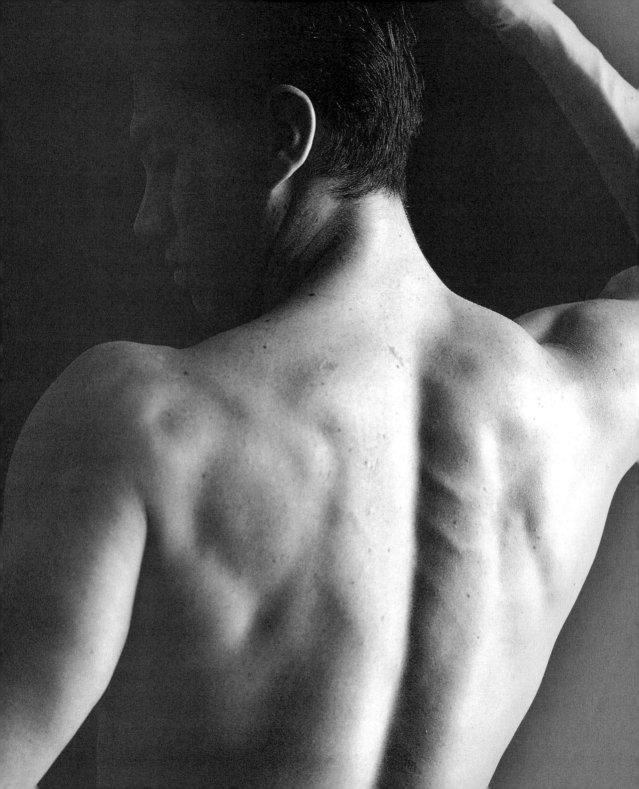

Part two Treating common conditions

● ● ● ● ● ● ● ● ● ● ● ● ●

The following pages will show you how to use magnets to relieve many common ailments including migraine, cramp, arthritis and muscle strain. By using the information on the meridian points given on pages 20–32 together with the illustrations given here specific to each condition, you will be able to use magnets to heal yourself and others. Each section contains general facts and advice on detecting and treating a common condition, followed by detailed information illustrating how to use magnets for pain relief and healing. You will also find advice on when to use magnets to heal and which alternative therapies can be used in conjunction with magnets.

Each condition is also illustrated with one, or more, case histories from real life, which show how magnets can be used to heal and improve our everyday lives.

● ● ● ● ● ● ● ● ● ● ● ● ●

Using magnets for health

Suppliers of small magnets used in healthcare promote their products for the relief of muscular stiffness and tension. Our modern intoxication with litigation and seeking to blame others for our own failure to use common sense has led suppliers, and even writers, to be very cautious when suggesting therapeutic uses for magnets. The opposition of the medical establishment and pharmaceutical industry to the idea that people could treat themselves effectively with inexpensive and non-chemical methods of healthcare has fuelled this caution.

Only use magnets externally and do not allow children to play with them. Apply common sense, follow the general directions given in this book and your experience of using small magnets will be safe and – in about eighty per cent of cases – beneficial.

Use your magnets to seek relief from pain. The following pages suggest how magnets can be used to deal with a variety of specific painful symptoms.

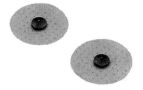

Consult your doctor

Persistent pain or ill-health is not normal, and the advice of your medical practitioner should always be sought in such cases. Holistic therapies are based on the general objective of removing the cause of ill-health as well as alleviating the symptoms. The relief of pain through magnet therapy, for example, may be a long-term program while the cause of pain is researched and dealt with, but it is always worthwhile.

If you are in any doubt about the compatibility of magnet therapy with another form of medical treatment that may be suitable for your condition, consult your medical practitioner. You should never change a chemical medication regime without first checking with the prescribing doctor; many modern chemical medications have design parameters that make it inadvisable for a patient to suddenly stop or change the doses prescribed.

Sprains and strains

Sprains and strains will benefit from the immediate application of magnetic bandages (bandages with magnetic material bonded into the fabric). The application of hot and cold compresses can also help. If you decide to use compresses, do so before placing the magnetic materials – bandages or a circle of small adhesive magnets – in place. When you have finished compress treatment, dry the skin before applying magnets. Remember that heat increases the blood flow, so hot compresses should not be applied to torn muscles which need a reduced blood flow in order to heal.

Other uses for magnets

Magnet therapy can also be used for less specific and obvious problems, more organic conditions that occur without specific injury and areas of pain. Identify the areas of tightest muscular tension in your body and use magnets to reduce this tension. For treatment of problems caused by a reduction in the performance of body organs, magnet therapy can be used in conjunction with other complementary therapies such as acupuncture, reflexology and shiatsu. Seek advice from your principal therapist and use the magnets on the acupuncture points to gain additional relief between your therapy sessions.

Magnet therapy should not adversely affect treatment with other medicinal therapies such as homeopathy, herbal medicine or therapies such as shiatsu or reflexology. In fact, some tests indicate the dual-therapy approach gives results greater than the sum of the two separate therapies. Magnets, however, should not be allowed to come into contact with homeopathic medicines, aromatherapy oils and strong scents or flavors, as they may have an adverse reaction on them.

Warning

In cases of obvious injury, such as sports injuries, follow the simple rule that magnets will improve blood flow and therefore should be used only if there is absolutely no bleeding, internally or externally. A torn muscle will benefit from magnets but only once the possibility of internal bleeding has passed (usually four to five days after the injury).

Migraine

A migraine is more than a bad headache. A migraine sufferer is effectively disabled for the duration of an attack and may have to remain totally inactive until it passes. In addition to a headache, which can affect just one side of the head (but is more usually all over), there is often a loss of vision, sickness and dizziness. Many people experience zigzag flashes of light that impair their vision.

Migraine triggers

Experience has shown that there are three basic migraine triggers: intolerance of certain types of food; stress; and hormone cycles. Individuals may have different trigger levels to any or all of the above. For many people, it is the combination of factors that causes the problem and this combination is not always the same, meaning that the actual cause can vary from migraine to migraine.

Preventative treatment

If you suspect your migraines are triggered by certain foods, cut them out of your diet to see whether there is any improvement.

Research in the US has indicated that sufferers of migraines and headaches brought on by stress should rub the part of the neck between the base of the skull and the first spinal vertebra, to ease tension in a small muscle called the Rectus capitis posterior minor.

Many people experience muscular tension in the upper back and shoulders, particularly between the shoulder blade and the spine, before and during an attack. Most sufferers start to recognize their own early-warning signals. Application of magnets at this stage, together with practical relaxation techniques, helps reduce the symptoms of the migraine or even prevent it altogether. Treatment as early as possible is advised.

For women suffering from cyclical migraines, usually hormone-related, it is beneficial to keep a diary and start remedial action with magnets and relaxation twenty-four hours before an attack.

Using magnets for migraines

Research at the Koestler Foundation in the US has revealed the effects of extremely low-frequency electromagnetic energy on migraines. Patients were asked to continuously wear a small "generator" that provided electromagnetic stimulation. The results of the study showed a reduction in both pain levels and the frequency of attacks.

Earlier research work had shown that weak electrical forces induced in the brain modify the excitability of central neurons (cells that conduct nerve impulses), and that electro- magnetic fields can affect ionic levels across cell membranes. It was also proved that the electrical characteristics of body fluids change on exposure to such fields. More simply, this means that small electrical and magnetic forces can change the way the fluids in the body work. Many migraine sufferers describe their attacks in electrical terms. The description of an electrical storm in the head is common, and with a proven link between magnetism and electrical activity, the basis for using magnets in the treatment of migraine is established.

Reducing migraine pain with small magnets

As soon as you get the first early-warning signal of an impending attack, adhere the magnets in place with the north pole touching the skin, on the upper back between the shoulder blades (you may need some help reaching this area), on the top of the feet and on the head. For more detailed instructions, refer to the illustrations and specific locations described in the case examples on the following pages.

In all cases, fix the magnet with the north pole touching the skin. To make sure you have the correct acupuncture point, apply gentle pressure in the area described and find the tender spot, then fix the magnets accordingly. Leave the magnets in place until all symptoms or danger signals have passed. Painkillers and any other treatments can be used at the same time. Try to relax. If a hot or warm bath helps, apply the magnets after drying off thoroughly.

Tension and stress-related migraines

Apply magnets to the acupuncture points described below, using the meridian illustrations on pages 24–32 to help you.

Between points B 14 and B 43 Between the shoulder blade and spine, just above the center of the shoulder blades.

Between points B 16 and B 45 Between the shoulder blade and spine, about 2–5 cm (6–2 in) above the bottom of the shoulder blade.

SI 14 The top of the shoulder blade, about 2 cm (1 in) from the top of the shoulder blade on the spine side.

T 15 On the back of the shoulder above the shoulder blade (still on the back), about midway between the center of the spine and the outer tip of the shoulder).

GB 21 About 2 cm (1 in) above T 15.

GB 12 Below and behind the ear on the back of the head.

B 10 In the hollow at the base of the skull where the neck joins the head.

Liv 3 On the feet between the big toe and the next one, about 2–5 cm (1–2 in) up from the web between the toes (see page 32).

LI 4 On the back of the hands, between the thumb and first finger at the "V" formed by the bones where the thumb separates from the rest of the fingers.

GB 1 On the face outside the eye at the outer "corner" of the eye.

On the face **between the ear and the eye**, about one-third of the way up the ear and about halfway across towards the eye.

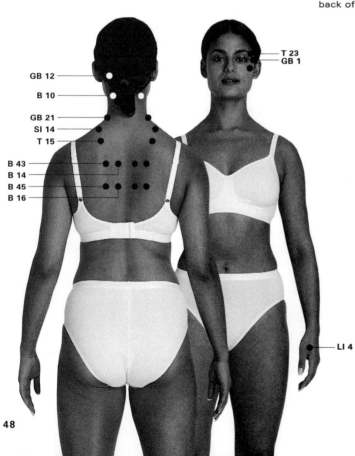

GB 12
B 10
GB 21
SI 14
T 15
B 43
B 14
B 45
B 16
T 23
GB 1
LI 4

Food intolerance-related migraines

Apply magnets to the points described below.

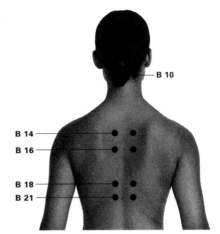

St 36 On the outside of the leg just below the knee (see page 29).

Liv 3 On the feet between the big toe and the next one, about 2–5 cm (1–2 in) up from the web between the toes (see page 32).

LI 4 On the back of the hands, between the thumb and first finger at the "V" formed by the bones where the thumb separates from the rest of the fingers (see left).

K 1 Under the foot on the center line of the sole and just behind the ball of the toes (see page 28).

B 18 On the back next to the spine, about halfway between the bottom of the shoulder blade and the bottom floating rib.

B 21 On the back next to the spine, just below the point where the last rib attaches to the spine.

B 10 In the hollow at the base of the skull where the neck goes into the head.

GB 1 On the face outside the eye at the outer "corner" of the eye.

T 23 Just above GB 1. **Between points B 14 and B 43** and **between points B 16 and B 45**, as described for tension and stress-related migraines.

MIGRAINE

Name: **Mary**   Age: **43**

Symptoms

Mary was suffering from disabling migraines twice a month lasting three days.

Treatment

Massage of the back and upper neck revealed areas of muscular tension and tightness. Acupuncture during the severe part of an attack gave some short-term relief. For subsequent attacks, as soon as the first early-warning signs manifested themselves, magnets were applied to the points shown for stress- and tension-related migraines, and left in place for five days. Mary experienced a less severe migraine than usual. The same procedure was carried out with the next five attacks. On each occasion the severity of the migraine lessened until Mary experienced no more than a mild headache. Magnets were then left in place for seven days on **Liv 3**, **LI 4** and **T 15**. Mary now has less severe migraines only once a year. Magnets may still be used at the onset of a migraine to reduce even further any adverse effects.

Circulation problems and cramp

Circulation problems occur when the circulation of blood in the blood vessels is reduced; this is easier to notice when there is a reduced blood flow to a specific area of the body. Poor circulation can be indicated by a variety of symptoms, including numbness, tingling or cramp, which is the prolonged, painful contraction of a muscle. Although cramp can be caused by an imbalance of the salts in the body, it is more often a result of fatigue, bad posture or stress. Cramp is also defined as a spasm in the muscles, which makes it impossible to perform a specific task, but allows the use of these muscles for any other movement. Improving the blood flow to a cramped muscle will speed up the movement of salts and overcome the adverse effects of whatever caused the spasm in the first place.

Diet and exercise

The quality of the blood, the ability of the blood vessels to convey blood around the body and the efficiency of the heart are all very much influenced by diet and exercise. All circulation disorders need to be checked out by a medical practitioner and a review of diet and exercise regimes undertaken. Smoking and heavy drinking should be avoided. However many magnets are applied to a body, they will be of no use if the cause of the problem is continually reintroduced.

Common causes of cramp

Cramp often occurs during the night with the sufferer being woken by severe pain in the lower leg or foot. Returning blood flow often induces the "pins and needles" sensation or unpleasant tingling feeling in the affected part of the body. This type of cramp is often due to the elevation (relative to the heart) of the limbs while in a relaxed state, which causes a drop in the pressure that drives blood around that lower limb.

Warning

Always seek medical advice if you have severe pain and disability, particularly if you suspect that these are related to circulation disorders.

Sports and fitness enthusiasts, both amateur and professional, can suffer from cramp if they fail to warm up or cool down correctly and, sometimes, if they make excessive demands on the circulation system. Excessive sweating, which reduces the levels of salt in the body, can also cause cramp. Such salt loss can be due to over-exercise or being in a climate that is much hotter than the body is used to.

Mechanical causes of cramp

Car drivers who have to sit in the same position for long periods with the edge of the seat pressing against the back of the lower thigh may also experience cramp, which can be dangerously distracting if the pain is severe. This form of cramp is caused by mechanical pressure stopping the blood flow, and is not a physiological disorder.

Placing the magnets

Blood is pumped around the body by the heart. Instructions are generally given to place the magnets above the site of reduced circulation, which means nearer to the heart in the blood flow system. For problems in the lower leg, place the magnets above the knee (as shown, right); for problems in the lower arm, place the magnets above the elbow. As a general rule, place the magnets between the pain area and the heart.

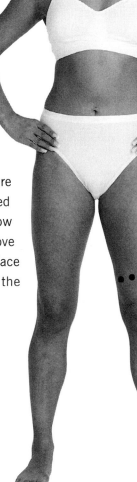

Other therapies

Treatments which successfully augment magnet therapy for circulation problems are:

- Yoga
- Shiatsu
- Gentle exercise

CRAMP

Name: **Catherine**   Age: **78**

Symptoms

Catherine was being woken more often than usual with cramp. It transpired that she had suffered from intermittent night-time cramp in her lower right leg for a number of years. A check on Catherine's diet and level of exercise indicated that both were reasonable for her age.

It is quite usual for patients with chronic conditions to have very little precise information about when a condition starts and what preceding events, if any, may have triggered it. In such cases, the therapist must deal with the situation without any real knowledge of the cause.

Treatment

Catherine did not want a visible circle of adhesive tape around her leg, so small magnets of around 600 gauss each were applied above her hemline, about 8 cm (3 in) **above the right knee** and spaced at 5 cm (2 in) intervals. Within two days, she announced that she had not had cramp since the magnets were put on. The magnets were removed after five days and Catherine has not suffered from cramp in the six months since treatment.

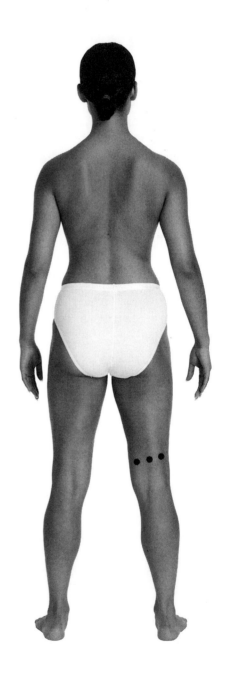

NUMB ARM AND HAND

Name: **Christopher**   Age: **49**

Symptoms

Christopher was suffering a numbness in the left arm and hand. His medical practitioner had described the condition as a reduced tactile sensation in the lower left arm and hand. He had advised rest and anti-depressants.

Christopher's blood pressure was within acceptable levels and although his cholesterol levels were a little high, they were not excessive. He did not smoke, had never been really ill and his alcohol intake was not extreme. His diet and physical activity levels were not good, although they were normal for a busy business executive with a family. Christopher was right-handed and had to drive many miles a week in his car, which had a manual, left-handed gear change. His general stress level was high, but not dangerously so.

Treatment

A course of five shiatsu treatments was started, with magnet therapy conducted in between. To prevent stress-related problems in the longer-term, Christopher was advised to take up yoga, to be more careful with his diet and to walk more – an hour's walk in the country can often undo much of the harm of a week's stress.

Magnets were placed on the left arm only. The positions used were: **LI 15** the "point" of the left shoulder; **GB 21** on top of the shoulder about halfway between the

neck and the point of the arm; and **LI 4** on the back of the hands between the thumb and first finger at the "V" formed by the bones where the thumb separates from the rest of the fingers. Further magnets were placed in a circle about 8 cm (3 in) **above the elbow** at intervals of 5 cm (2 in).

Christopher reported a very gradual improvement in his condition, and, after the fifth shiatsu treatment, had no numbness at all. His general stress levels also seemed to have decreased.

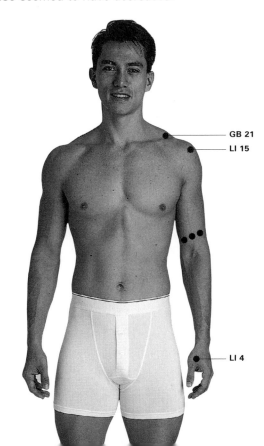

GB 21

LI 15

LI 4

Sports injuries

Major sports injuries need specialist medical attention. If you are in any doubt at all about the severity of an injury, seek immediate qualified help. Head injuries – or even suspected head injuries – should be treated by fully qualified medical specialists as soon as possible after an accident. Do not take risks with injuries; they can be much worse than they initially appear.

Minor sports injuries also need immediate attention if they are to be resolved quickly and not turn into chronic problems. The long-term postural problems of many people stem from relatively minor injuries that were not given the correct attention at the right time.

To cover all possible types of sports injury would take an exhaustive specialist book, but to use magnet therapy as an aid to self-help, I have focused on the more common and less serious types of problem.

Strains and sprains

Strains and sprains are the most common sports injuries, resulting from the overstretching of the tissue that connects muscles to bones or connects bone to bone around a moveable joint. This overstretching is usually the result of the sudden and unexpected change of the direction of load (the combination of body weight and the weight of whatever is being lifted) on the area which ends up damaged. It is the change of direction rather than actual load itself that causes this type of damage. The application of alternating hot and cold compresses, and the use of massage and magnet therapy will all help these injuries to heal.

Torn muscles

A sudden increase in the actual load can be the cause of more serious problems, such as

---

Warning

Do not use magnets where bleeding – internal or external – is taking place. This is because severed capillaries and blood vessels need a reduced blood flow and restricted local blood pressure in order to heal. Magnets will produce the opposite effect.

torn and ruptured muscles or connecting tissues. The application of cold compresses is the best immediate action to take, and expert care and advice is vital. Massage and magnets should be avoided until all internal bleeding has stopped. Seriously torn muscles involving the rupture of large amounts of tissue, or small amounts of vital tissue, are very serious and will take a long time to heal fully. Repaired tissue will never be as strong as the original material and so sites of previous injury are at risk from damage.

Prevention

Minor injuries can be prevented by increased flexibility, which can be achieved through yoga and other forms of suppleness training. Being aware of the causes of injury will also help. Practical jokes in a gym are dangerous. Loss of temper on the sports field can result in injuries way beyond the expected consequence. Failure to focus on what you are doing can have very painful results. Take care, and everyone can enjoy pain-free sporting activity.

Treatment with small magnets

The basic aim is to bring nutrients and repair materials to the damaged site, and to remove waste products. Magnets are positioned to improve blood flow, reduce swelling and ease pain. Place a small magnet at the center of the damaged area and additional magnets all around it, at spaces of about 5 cm (2 in). The illustration, left, shows magnet positions for damage to a shoulder, with magnets placed on the source of the pain and the surrounding area. For an injury to a limb (such as the left wrist, as shown here), place magnets in a circle around the limb between the injury and the heart. The magnet shown on the hand can also be used for wrist pain (see page 57).

Golf injuries

Many well-known professional golfers use magnets, magnetic bandages and mattresses with magnets in place to ease the discomfort of injuries, caused by a combination of the overuse of particular joints and/or muscle tissue, as well as prolonged exposure to the cold, wet and wind.

Magnetic bandages have been credited with helping many cases of "golfing elbow." A small magnet placed on **LI 15** the "point" of the right shoulder and **LI 4** (see page 53), on the back of the hand at the "V" formed by the bone of the thumb meeting the carpal bone next to it, will also speed up recovery. The problem for most professional sports people is that relatively small injuries that would benefit from rest are ignored and the activity is pursued, regardless of pain. Magnets allow the activity to be continued, at the same time providing a form of treatment.

Golf players, and all racket game players, can also suffer from inflammation of the pectoral muscle at the point where it "inserts" (attaches) into the humerus (upper bone in the arm). Pain and weakness occur when the upper arm is drawn towards the chest against resistance. Magnets placed all around the affected area of the upper arm and the front of the shoulder will speed recovery.

Racket sports

Inflamed shoulder muscles cause pain during exertion and aches after exertion. If an examination has taken place to ensure that a muscle has not been torn, the magnets can then be applied (as shown in the illustration on page 55) to the center of the tenderest spot, determined by gentle pressure, and then in a circle around the aching area.

Other therapies

Treatments which successfully augment magnet therapy for sports injuries are:

• Traction and manipulation when recommended by a medical practitioner

• Massage

WRIST PAIN

Name: **Robert**   Age: **28**

Symptoms

Robert, a javelin thrower, reported pain and loss of mobility in his right wrist; the condition had worsened over the last few days but there was no visible discoloration or swelling.

Treatment

Magnets were placed on **LI 15** (the "point" of the right shoulder) and **around the wrist**, about 5 cm (2 in) above the wrist crease, at 2 cm (1 in) intervals. An additional magnet was adhered to **LI 4** (on the back of the hand, at the "V" formed by the bone of the thumb meeting the carpal bone next to it – see page 55.)

Robert was advised to stop throwing for a week, but he was allowed to lightly exercise the arms and do gentle running and walking. After ten days, he reported some reduction in pain but a return to full loading had caused discomfort. A magnetic bandage was placed around the wrist to give physical support to the area. Although Robert still uses this support when training or competing, he otherwise has full mobility.

TOE INJURY

Name: **Stephanie**   Age: **24**

Symptoms

Stephanie had run barefoot into an immovable object and badly hurt the small toe of her right foot. She was in great pain but after eighteen hours of rest there was no swelling or discoloration that would indicate internal bleeding.

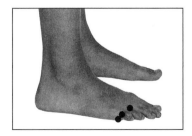

Treatment

Magnets were applied to the **base of the toe, on the outside edge of the foot** and to the **web on top of the foot** between the small toe and its neighbor. After two days the pain had reduced and after four days the magnets were removed. A further seven days of relative rest were recommended, after which cautious exercise was allowed, with the toe protected with adhesive tape wound around the foot to prevent the small toe from spreading and becoming dislocated. After a further seven days, Stephanie was able to resume her normal keep-fit regime.

Menstrual problems

The blood and other material discharged from the uterus at the time of menstruation are called the menses. The normal duration of this discharge is from three to seven days, occurring at four-week intervals. These basic facts give no hint to the amount of pain and discomfort some women experience before and during bleeding. But in addition to the physical pain, some women also experience hormone-influenced mood swings and nervous tension.

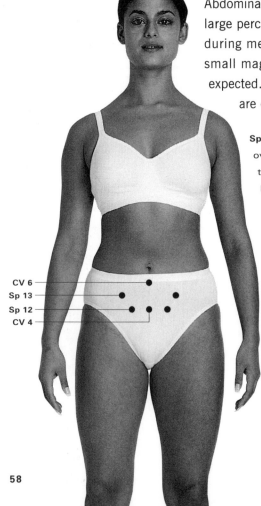

Abdominal cramps

Abdominal pains, generally referred to as cramps, occur in a very large percentage of women just before the onset of bleeding and during menstruation. These pains can be reduced by adhering small magnets to selected points the day before the pains are expected. Apply magnets to these selected points, most of which are on both sides of the body:

Sp 12 On the front of the body over the pelvic bone where the ball of the hip joint is located in the pelvic girdle.
Sp 13 Just above and outside Sp 12.
B 27 Either side of the spine, just below the last flexible vertebrae (see right).

B 28 2 cm (1 in) below B 27 (see right).

Also beneficial are **CV 6** (on the center line of the front of the body, just below an imaginary line drawn across the top of the hip bones, or pelvic girdle) and **CV 4** (about 5 cm or 2 in directly below CV 6).

CV 6
Sp 13
Sp 12
CV 4

Other therapies

Treatments which successfully augment magnet therapy for menstrual problems are:

• Yoga
• Relaxation techniques
• Painkillers taken under supervision
• Shiatsu

In some cases, benefit may be obtained by placing magnets on:

B 48 On the back, either side of the line of the spine about midway out from the center line to the edge of the body.

Sp 6 About 5 cm (2 in) above the ankle bone, just behind the shin bone (see page 60). Do not use this point if pregnancy is a possibility and the cramps are caused by pregnancy rather than menstruation.

Sp 4 On the inside edge of the foot about halfway between the heel and the big toe on the bony ridge that can be felt along this edge (see page 60).

Lower-back pain

Many women suffer lower-back pain during their cycle. Use the following points on both sides of the body (they are shown on the right-hand side of the body in this illustration):

B 29 and **B 30** Either side of the center line on the back, level with the hip socket and about 2 cm (1 in) from the center line.

Sp 12 See page 58.

B 23 and **B 25** Either side of the center line of the back. B 25 is just below the top of the hip structure and B 23 is just above it (see right).

Premenstrual syndrome

PMS (or PMT) is the term usually used when referring to the emotional stress and nervous tension experienced before menstruation. To help with PMS, apply magnets to:

B 31 and **B 32** Both points are just either side of the center line of the back, just below B 27 (B 32 is below B 31); **CV 6**, **CV 4** (see left), **B 48** (see above) and **Sp 4** (see page 60).

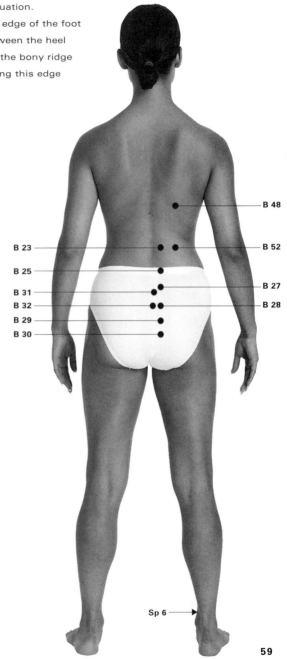

B 48

B 23

B 52

B 25

B 27

B 31

B 32

B 28

B 29

B 30

Sp 6

Irregular periods

If your cycle is erratic and unpredictable, a very thorough medical examination should be carried out to ensure that all the systems of the body are working as they should. If you are given the all clear, and taking the birth control pill is not an option for regulating the cycle, then magnets can be used for ten days every month, starting on the day after the period stops, on **CV 6**, **CV 4** and **Sp 6**.

Nausea

For cases of nausea, the most advantageous place to put a magnet is on the inside of the wrist at **P 6**. This is about 5 cm (2 in) up from the wrist crease on the center line of the arm between the two blood vessels.

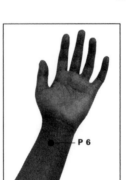

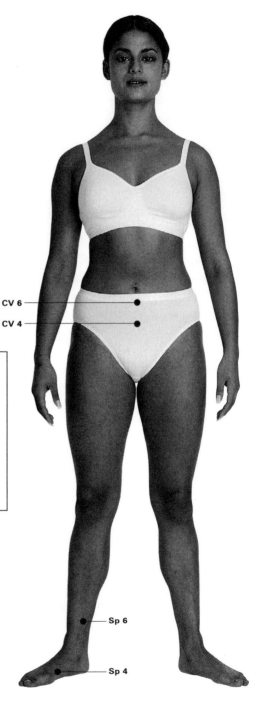

Warning

Do not use point **Sp 6** if there is any likelihood that the person you are treating may be pregnant.

ABDOMINAL CRAMPS

Name: **Diane**   Age: **20**

Symptoms

Diane suffered from a severe and disabling cramp that lasted for five days every cycle, when she was forced to go to bed with a hot-water bottle. Her doctor had recommended strong analgesic painkillers, but she was reluctant to take these on a long-term basis. The condition had been present since puberty, affecting school, exam results, college attendance, and so on. Diane had tried a few alternative treatments, each providing some improvement in the short term. However, the cost of ongoing therapy was a big concern, and she wished to find a way she could improve her life for herself.

Treatment

As for all treatments, the three stages to be considered are the initial coping strategy, therapy and change. For Diane, the coping strategy was painkillers and the therapy was the application of magnets before the expected attack of cramps. But the last stage – that of change – was much more problematic as, in this case, the therapy was simply another coping strategy since real change could only come about through pregnancy or the passing of time.

Small magnets were applied, as shown for abdominal cramps on page 58, and left in place until one day after the cramps had gone. After the treatment had been used for several months, Diane reported that the application of the magnets usually reduced the levels of pain sufficiently to allow her to live a normal life without painkillers. However, if a day occurred when the pain was too much to bear, then both painkillers and magnets could be used together.

LOWER-BACK PAIN

Name: **Elaine**   Age: **25**

Symptoms

Elaine complained of lower-back pain that had only recently started to aggravate her. She was not pregnant and did not wish to be. It was determined that the pain was associated with her menstrual cycle and, while it was not severe enough for her to consult her medical practitioner, it was, nevertheless, still a problem to her.

Treatment

Magnets were fixed to the body in the positions described for lower-back pain on page 59.

Elaine reused these at the first onset of the pain, keeping them in place until her period was over. The reduction in pain allowed her to follow her normal routine without painkillers.

Back pain

Statistics about back pain indicate that it is the cause of more time off work, more misery and more discomfort than practically anything else. What causes it? Why don't we evolve stronger backs? How do we prevent the problem, and how do we resolve it?

Analyzing back pain

There are three main types of back pain: muscular, skeletal and organ-related, each with a huge range of causes and effects. Diagnosis of the *cause* of back pain is vital if the problem is to be alleviated, and if the cause is serious illness, such as cancer, it must be treated by appropriately qualified medical practitioners. There has been some research using strong electromagnetic fields to "treat" cancer, but as yet it is an unproven technique.

Using magnets for back pain

It would take thousands of years to evolve stronger backs that are better adapted to our lifestyles. Until then, as a general guide, magnet therapy can be used to help with a variety of back conditions. These can range from muscular back pain, postural distortions (these can be helped in conjunction with physical manipulation work such as osteopathy, chiropractic or shiatsu massage), impact injuries, temporary enforced postural distortion, and (to a lesser extent) deterioration due to age.

Back pain caused by pregnancy can be relieved by magnets. They can help ease the discomfort caused to the back by the changes in weight and balance that pull muscles and joints out of place.

Impact injuries can also benefit from the use of small magnets, once it has been established that no internal injury or broken bones have been sustained.

> **Warning**
> Before treating back pain yourself, see your medical practitioner.

Distortion of the skeletal structure due to bad posture will cause back pain. Alleviating this pain has to be seen as a long-term process. The first step is to ensure that the posture is improved. This may result in the pain increasing temporarily as muscles accustomed to a certain position are forced back to their correct position.

A less obvious cause of back pain is a disturbance of the balance between the relative strengths of the back muscles: those that pull us upright and backwards, and those counteracting muscles in the abdomen and chest, which hold the back muscles in balance. If either becomes relatively too strong for the other, then distortion and back pain may result.

Exercising

Simply lying down flat on the floor and letting the spine settle will often help. The standard recovery position for back pain is to lie on the floor on your back with your lower legs up on a chair parallel to the floor, your back flat on the floor and your thighs at a ninety-degree angle to the floor.

Other therapies

Treatments which successfully augment magnet therapy for back pain are:

• Chiropractic techniques

• Osteopathy

• Massage

• Shiatsu

• Painkillers under supervision

• Supervised yoga and other stretching exercises

Locating back pain

Back pain and backache are usually very difficult to pinpoint. The exact location of the center of the problem is difficult to determine and it may shift around, depending on the posture and weight distribution at the time it is being described. Placing small magnets around the general area of discomfort will help. If the center of the pain can be located, place a magnet on this spot, too. Using magnetic bandages or wraps to surround the whole lower back will be beneficial, but ensure that the magnetic parts of the bandage are on the back.

LOWER-BACK PAIN

Name: **David**   Age: **28**

Symptom

David came to the clinic with a common complaint: lower-back pain. He did not know why he should be experiencing such discomfort or how he could have injured himself. He was reasonably fit, and his diet and activity levels were adequate. A physical examination eliminated the possibility of kidney problems, but it did indicate muscular tension and rigidity rather than a displacement of the bones.

David's posture while working gave a clue to the possible cause: his job was demanding and pressurized, and the height of his chair in relation to his desk caused the lower back muscles to be stretched while he was under "mental" stress or tension.

Treatment

David was shown how to do the easy "cat and dog" exercises (see below). These exercises flex all the back without putting too much strain on any particular area. He was also advised to keep warm at all times and not allow his posture to become fixed in any one position. Magnets were fixed in the following positions: **either side of the spine**, about 2 cm (1 in) either side of the center line, at the point where the spine starts to be flexible; **in a circle just above the pelvic girdle** around the first magnets, at a distance of about 10 cm (4 in). David reported an improvement the next day, and within six days he was experiencing only slight twinges of pain.

Cat and dog exercises

1 *Get on to your hands and knees with your head and back parallel to the floor.*

2 *Arch your head up and abdomen down into "dog pose."*

3 *Move smoothly into "cat pose" by arching your neck down and drawing your abdomen up away from the floor. Your back is now arched upwards. Rock back and forward again and return to the original position. Repeat the two movements several times, slowly.*

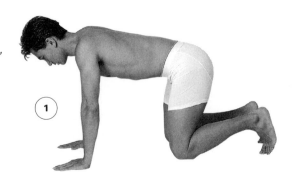

PAIN BETWEEN SHOULDER BLADES

Name: **Janet** Age: **35**

Symptoms

Janet was experiencing severe stiffness and discomfort in the upper back. She was physically active, materially comfortable and had a healthy diet and lifestyle. There were no known injuries that could be held responsible for the problem. Examination showed muscular tension between the lower parts of the shoulder blades. She did not suffer from headaches. Discussion revealed that Janet carried an emotional burden which she felt was imposed on her by others.

Treatment

Experience has shown that we physically carry the emotional tension that we generate inside ourselves in the muscles at the top of the shoulder blades, and that the emotional tension generated from outside ourselves is carried between the lower parts of the shoulder blades. Accordingly, magnets were placed **in lines either side of the spine**, between the spine and the shoulder blades, starting 5 cm (2 in) below the lowest point of the shoulder blade and going up to the top of the shoulder blade and about 5 cm (2 in) apart. Janet was advised to take up yoga and develop physical relaxation techniques. There was improvement within two days and, gradually, the stiffness and discomfort were reduced. In addition, the release of the locked-in tension allowed Janet to deal with the issues that had caused the problem in the first place.

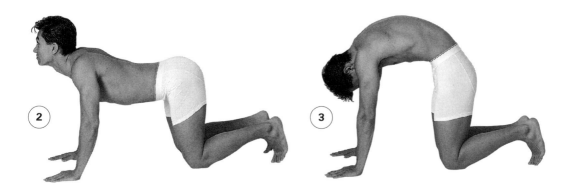

② ③

Rheumatism

Rheumatism is the name given to any disorder in which the muscles and joints are afflicted by aches and pains, so it could be said that many of us suffer from temporary rheumatism quite often!

Rheumatoid arthritis

Rheumatoid arthritis is a particular form of arthritis which, unless held in check by treatment, progressively reduces the amount of pain-free movement in the joints. Usually starting in the fingers, wrists and ankles, it can spread to the hips, knees and shoulders. X-rays and blood tests can show changes around the affected joints indicating the presence of rheumatoid arthritis. This can be a serious, debilitating illness, and medical attention is vital to treat it.

Muscular aches and pains

Although aches and pains in the muscles do not usually cause disablement, they are uncomfortable and troublesome. Magnets do help relieve these pains quite effectively, and if the cause can be identified and treated, there will be a dramatic improvement in the enjoyment of life.

It is not necessary to know the shape, position and action of each muscle to deal with minor discomfort, but if severe pain or repeated problems occur, it is wise to seek professional help. If your medical practitioner can only prescribe painkillers, consult a masseur, aromatherapist or shiatsu practitioner. Help yourself by examining your lifestyle, posture and physical activities, and check to see if you are repeatedly inflicting the condition on yourself. When we are not engaged in physical activity, and especially if we are under stress, we are likely to make some muscles position themselves badly, for example when we hunch our shoulders over a computer keyboard.

Warning

If the pain persists, recurs or is severe, seek medical attention.

Diet and rheumatism

Many books have been written and studies undertaken which indicate that a change in diet will improve the chances of preventing, or recovery from, rheumatism or arthritis (see pages 70–71). Food intolerance can present itself as muscular pain. An intolerance of a food that was previously "safe" can develop; it is not always apparent that our bodies have a problem with any particular chemical combination from the first taste of a food containing those chemicals. But because human beings are so different from each other, and because there is an almost infinite range of food combinations available, it is practically impossible to give general dietary advice to suit everyone.

Ageing and rheumatism

As we get older, we become less supple. The accumulation of minor injuries over the years starts to have an effect. Reduced levels of activity, reduced suppleness and the accumulation of damaged tissue all result in a less efficient blood flow. This means that the waste products from muscular activity are not removed as well as they were in our youth, and the sudden burst of seasonal physical activity we subject ourselves to, such as gardening, leaves residues of by-product waste in our muscles, resulting in stiffness and pain. Post-activity hot baths, gradually increasing the amount of exercise, together with magnet therapy, can all help alleviate the discomfort.

Relieving rheumatic pain

Magnets have been found to be very beneficial in the treatment and relief of general rheumatic pains. Whether they are used instead of painkillers or in conjunction with them, they still provide considerable benefit to most people. Place the magnets around the area of pain and in the center of it. Try to relax and keep the body warm.

Other therapies

Treatments which successfully augment magnet therapy for rheumatic pain are:

- Massage
- Yoga
- Warmth
- Shiatsu

SHOULDER AND UPPER-THIGH PAIN

CASE HISTORY

Name: **Geoffrey**   Age: **66**

Symptoms

Geoffrey asked if there was anything that could be done about the pains in his shoulders and upper thighs. He had recently retired from his job as a truck driver and now devoted himself to gardening. Although these increased activities required a little more bending of the legs and manipulation of the fingers than he had been used to, gardening was not something new, as he had always enjoyed it. Geoffrey's all-round muscle tone was good, and his upper arms were particularly strong. His diet had been too high in fatty foods for many years but this had improved since retirement.

Treatment

Geoffrey was advised to increase his general physical activity level by joining a gym or taking up a sport. He was also encouraged to walk a mile a day. Simple stretching exercises were devised to improve his posture.

Small magnets were placed on the **"point" of each shoulder; in the middle of each shoulder blade; either side of the spine**, about halfway down the shoulder blade, between the shoulder blade and the spine; and **on the trunk** of the body under the arm (not shown on the illustration); on **GB 31** (outside of the leg at a height where the longest finger would touch the seam of trousers if standing level and upright); in a circle **around each upper thigh**, about 8 cm (3 in) above GB 31.

Geoffrey reported some improvement after two days but initially found it difficult to keep the magnets in position. They were fixed with waterproof surgical tape for ten days. He found a great reduction in discomfort and improved mobility.

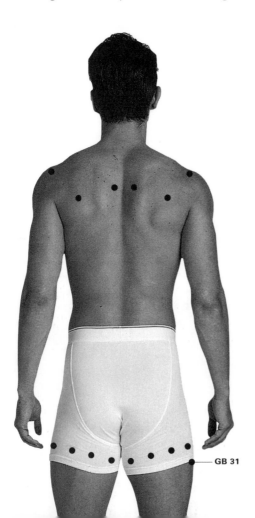

GB 31

HIP AND ARM PAIN

Name: **Rebecca**   Age: **51**

Symptoms

Rebecca came to the clinic with rheumatic pains in her hips and arms. She had been a very active tennis player all her life and resented the discomfort that had started to restrict her playing. She took painkillers every day. She had two adult children who lived away from home. The emotional and material aspects of her life were settled and comfortable. Her diet was well-balanced, with fresh foods predominating. She did not smoke and only drank alcohol in moderation.

Treatment

Rebecca was advised to walk at least a mile a day and to follow a course of shiatsu or aromatherapy. She was also encouraged to swim every week as this type of "no weight load" exercise is very good for general, non-disabling rheumatic problems, provided that the damp atmosphere does not cause any aggravation.

Magnets were placed on **GB 31**, as described left, and in circles **around the waist and the upper arms** (see illustration). Waterproof tape was used to keep the magnets in position for ten days, by which time Rebecca had been able to stop taking painkillers, although she did experience some minor withdrawal headaches for three days afterwards. Within a month, Rebecca's discomfort was greatly reduced and, subsequently,

her quality of life improved. Incidentally, she preferred shiatsu to aromatherapy massage and continued to have a "maintenance" treatment every month.

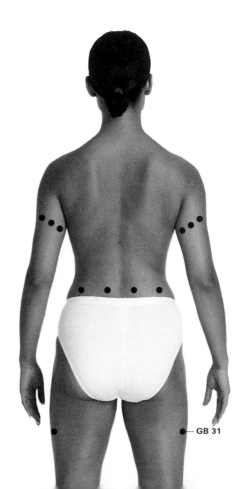

GB 31

Arthritis

Arthritis is the inflammation of one or more joints, characterized by swelling, warmth and redness of the overlying skin, pain and restricted movement. There are many possible causes, but the most common is the deterioration of tissue resulting from over-use and/or damage earlier in life. A great many people suffer from mild forms of arthritis and lead active lives, but severe forms of the condition can be totally disabling.

Osteoarthritis

In osteoarthritis, secondary changes occur to the underlying bone and in the cartilage of a joint. Relieving pressure across the joint reduces the load on the damaged structure and diminishes the discomfort and pain.

Osteoporosis

Osteoporosis is the loss of bony tissue that results in brittle bones which are liable to fracture. It can be a localized problem, caused by infection or injury affecting only a specific joint or bone, but it can be present throughout the body. HRT (hormone replacement therapy) does reduce the incidence of this disease in post-menopausal women, showing that changes in the body's chemistry influence the condition enormously.

Other therapies

Treatments which can successfully augment magnet therapy for arthritis are:

- Yoga
- Massage
- Shiatsu

Diet

Many people believe that fish oil, especially cod liver oil, in the diet will help reduce the impact of deterioration in cartilage and connective tissue caused by aging. Ginger and glucosamine as food supplements are also reported to be helpful. A diet containing sufficient amounts of fish oils and olive oil is important for everyone, but particularly for those living in damp and cold climates. It is better to try to ensure such a diet early in life rather than waiting until the pain gets noticeable and restrictive. However, it is never too late to start providing your body with beneficial supplements.

Magnets and arthritis

Severe arthritis is a crippling disease and it can occur in the very young. The repair of bone and connective tissue will not happen quickly, if at all, particularly in older sufferers, so do not expect a "cure" from magnet therapy. What magnets can do is help reduce the pain and improve the blood flow, thereby accelerating chemical re-building and the removal of waste products. They cannot, however, rebuild damaged tissue.

Magnets should be placed around the painful areas, generally encircling the most painful spot. For the legs and arms, it is best to place the magnets around the affected limb between the pain and the heart, as for cramp (as the illustration, left, shows for the right arm and left leg). Magnets should not adversely affect the use of HRT, whichever system of administration is involved.

Avoiding arthritis

The likelihood of suffering arthritis may be reduced by eating a good diet, maintaining flexibility through exercise and caring for injuries – all continuous processes in our lives. Using magnets will help damaged tissue rebuild itself and limit the long-term damage that can result in arthritis.

Warning

If you have raised blood pressure, only use magnets under expert supervision, and stop using magnets immediately should your blood pressure rise still further.

ARTHRITIC WRISTS AND FOREARMS

Name: **Peter**   Age: **45**

Symptoms

Peter complained of pain in his wrists and forearms, and was shocked when his doctor told him he had arthritis because he did not believe that someone of "his age" could suffer from it. Discussion revealed that Peter had been involved in a motor-cycle accident when he was twenty-three and had broken both wrists, which had healed well. He worked as an industrial sales engineer, which involved a lot of driving and typing.

Treatment

Since Peter had once broken his wrists, 1,000-gauss magnets were used to reach deep into the tissue of the body. They were fixed to **the "point" of each shoulder** and in a circle 2 cm (1 in) apart **around each arm**, about 2 cm (1 in) **above the wrist bone** (see illustration). They were left in place for seven days and some improvement in the level of pain was reported. The magnets were then removed for five days, before being replaced for an additional seven days. Again there was a reported improvement. This sequence of seven days with magnets and five days without was repeated five times. For the duration of the treatment, Peter took painkillers whenever he felt he needed them. At the end of the treatment, Peter announced that his pain had reduced so much that he was able to live normally without medication.

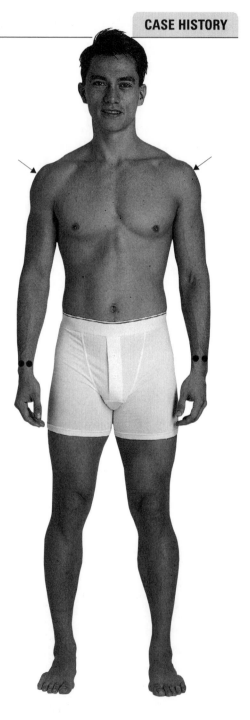

ARTHRITIC ANKLE, ARM, WRIST AND HAND   CASE HISTORY

Name: **George**   Age: **77**

Symptoms

George suffered pain in his left ankle, right arm, wrist and hand, which he had been told was due to arthritis. He also suffered from slightly raised blood pressure, for which he was taking medication. George agreed to try magnet therapy on the understanding that the magnets would be removed immediately if there were any signs of increased blood pressure.

Treatment

Magnets were first used in a circle **around the left leg**, about 5 cm (2 in) above the ankle bone. After five days, George was experiencing less pain. The magnets were removed and repositioned **around the right wrist**, about 5 cm (2 in) above the wrist bone. Again, the magnets were left in place for five days, after which there was a noticeable reduction in pain.

ARTHRITIC SHOULDER   CASE HISTORY

Name: **Valerie**   Age: **56**

Symptoms

Valerie came to the clinic as she had recently taken up golf but was getting pain in her left shoulder, which her medical practitioner put down to arthritis. Valerie was concerned as the pain restricted the amount of golf she could play, caused serious discomfort when it was cold and wet, and she was worried that the condition would worsen as she got older. She took analgesic painkillers on a daily basis, despite knowing that she would suffer withdrawal symptoms if she stopped taking them suddenly. Her mother had suffered from arthritis, but not until she was over seventy years old.

Treatment

Valerie's diet was discussed and she was advised to reduce the amount of stimulants (tea, coffee and alcohol) and dairy products that she regularly consumed.

A magnetic bandage was wrapped **around the affected shoulder** in the same pattern used by first-aiders for treating a broken shoulder, with the center of the bandage in the armpit of the injured side. This was kept in place for most of the first seven days of treatment, after which it was worn whenever she played golf. After a month, she reported reduced discomfort and more time on the golf course.

Sciatica

Sciatica is the name used to describe the intense pain felt down the back and outside of the thigh, leg and foot.

Causes of sciatica

Sciatica is usually caused by a damaged or degenerated disc of the spine. The discs in the spine act as cushions between the vertebrae, and if a disc cushioning lower vertebrae is damaged, the sciatic nerve (the body's longest nerve) is squashed as it leaves the channel running vertically down the center of the spine. This nerve transmits signals to the brain, indicating pain down the thigh and leg. The exact area of pain felt is dependent on which part of the sciatic nerve has been affected.

The onset of sciatic pain may be sudden and intense, and can be caused by lifting or twisting. In many instances, the condition is first caused by twisting under a load, even though the load may not be great – it is the combination of turning and the load that does the damage. Deterioration of a disc, which leads to sciatica, can be due to its continuous over-use, or to a malfunction in the individual's structural make-up. Degenerative diseases can also affect the area. As we get older, the slight deterioration of a disc caused by the body being unable to repair itself as quickly as it once did, coupled with our determination to physically act as we did when young, can result in sciatic pain.

Warning

Remember that although sciatic pain is felt in the legs, the damage is in the lower back and this is the area that should be treated with care and caution.

Terminology

Experts in sports medicine call damage to the disc between the third and fourth lumbar vertebrae "L4 syndrome"; damage between the fourth and fifth lumbar vertebrae "L5 syndrome"; and damage to the disc between the fifth lumbar vertebra and the first sacral vertebra "S1 syndrome."

The pain from L4 syndrome extends down the back of the thigh and over to the front of the knee. Pain from L5 syndrome goes down the outside of the thigh and leg, curving round to the front of the lower leg and down to the big toe. S1 syndrome affects the outside of the thigh and leg and extends to the small toe. The pain can be present in either or both legs, depending on the exact nature and extent of the damage to the affected disc.

Other therapies

Treatments which can successfully augment magnet therapy for sciatica are:

• Chiropractic treatment
• Gentle exercise and specific exercises
• Shiatsu
• Osteoporosis treatment
• Acupuncture

Establishing the cause of pain

It is essential to find out what has happened to cause the pain. Generalized pain in the lower back – lumbago – is not the same as sciatica and needs to be treated in a different way. Damage to vertebrae higher up the back also calls for different treatment. X-rays and scans will determine if there is any disc damage or degeneration. The cause and severity of the degeneration is very important to establish, just in case it is a problem that could, if left untreated, spread to other parts of the skeletal system.

Treating sciatica

Our aims when using magnets to treat sciatica are: to relieve pain and to try to improve the condition of the spine in the area that is causing the problem. Small magnets are placed in a line down the spine and in a circle around the area generally known as the lumbar region. Magnets can also be placed on both thighs at GB 31 (where the longest finger reaches if you stand upright).

GB 31

PAIN IN THIGHS

Name: **Timothy**   Age: **66**

Symptoms

Timothy, who had recently retired, called in at the clinic to ask if anything could be done for the pain he felt in both thighs. A consultation revealed that Timothy had assumed the pain was rheumatic and he had not consulted his medical practitioner, in the belief that nothing could be done to help. Further discussion revealed that Timothy had recently taken up golf and the pains had started to occur some time after a strenuous golfing holiday. Gentle pressure applied to the lower back, indicated tenderness. It was suggested that Timothy should ask his medical practitioner to refer him for an x-ray or scan, at the same time informing him that the problem was probably sciatic, caused by damage to the lower part of the spine, which put pressure on the nerve.

A week later, Timothy returned to the clinic with his x-rays showing slight damage to the area but not enough to cause very great problems. He had not played golf since his last visit and the pain had subsided. He asked if we could do anything that would enable him to resume his golf without the pain. Examination showed that the localized inflammation had reduced.

Treatment

Magnets were placed **around the tender area** and **on the spine** at the bottom of the back. It was not necessary to place magnets on the thighs. Timothy was advised to leave the magnets in place for five days, then have a series of massage and shiatsu sessions – alternating one week massage, the next shiatsu. After four weeks of such treatment, he should reapply the magnets for a further five days. During this time he could, and should take gentle exercise – preferably walking.

After six weeks, Timothy reported a considerable improvement. He did experience some discomfort but, by ensuring that his lower back was always covered and warm, having a weekly massage or shiatsu treatment, and being aware of the problem, he was able to enjoy playing golf. Whenever he felt any pain returning, he replaced the magnets.

HIP PAIN

Name: **Sarah**   Age: **73**

Symptoms

Sarah's medical practitioner had referred her to hospital for an x-ray after she reported pain in her hip. In the meantime, she came to the clinic in search of pain relief. Detailed questioning about the pain indicated that the sciatic nerve was involved, especially since she also had pain down her legs. She informed the radiographers of this when she was eventually seen at the hospital, but they would not x-ray anything other than her hip.

Treatment

While waiting for the x-ray appointment and the results, Sarah was treated with shiatsu, moxibustion (a traditional Chinese warming treatment that originally used burning moxa, but other materials can also be used, such as artemisia or plum wood) and massage. Magnets were placed **down the spine** and **in a circle around the lumbar area** and on the outside of both thighs at acupuncture point **GB 31** (where the longest finger reaches if you stand upright). The x-rays showed no damage to the hip, and the medical practitioner referred Sarah for further x-rays of the lower back. By that time, several weeks had passed and Sarah was feeling so much better that she cancelled the second x-ray appointment.

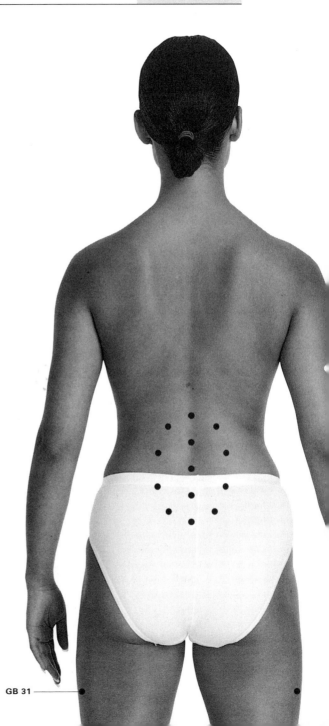

GB 31

Constipation

Constipation is the inability to empty the bowels or the difficult and painful emptying of them. Small, hard feces are also a sign of constipation. It is a distressing and painful condition that may indicate a very serious underlying problem.

The conventional treatment for constipation is with laxatives in the short-term and dietary changes – usually an increase in fiber – for the longer term. Dietary fiber, or roughage, is the part of food that cannot be digested or absorbed to provide energy. However, in some cases, too much fiber can cause problems.

The intestines

The bowels are also called the large intestine, and the colon is the main part of the large intestine. There are a number of different names for the same parts of the digestive system, which can cause confusion. The whole digestive system is often referred to as the gut. The colon is essentially a tube that reabsorbs water and substances called electrolytes from the undigested food that passes down its center. This food has come from the small intestine. At intervals, strong squeezing movements, called peristaltic movements, squeeze the now-dehydrated contents towards the rectum.

The colon is made up of the ascending colon, transverse colon, descending colon and the sigmoid colon – the end part just before the tube becomes the rectum. This, in turn, is just before the anus. Colonic irrigation, sometimes used to clean out the colon, is the washing-out of its contents with copious enemas, using either water or other medications.

Warning

If constipation lasts for more than four days or recurs frequently, consult your medical practitioner.

Causes of constipation

Constipation is mostly the uncomfortable symptom or side-effect of an existing health condition. Stress and anxiety are common causes, resulting in the abdominal wall muscles tightening, creating internal pressure on the system, which, in turn, disrupts the movements in the digestive system. Treatment of the stress will remedy the constipation without specifically treating the mechanics of digestion and the constipation.

Constipation can be caused by a variety of other things too: poor diet, which means that the food in the system clogs it up; degeneration of the colon; colon disease; failure of material to reach the colon, and so on.

The whole digestive process begins with chewed-up food in the mouth, which moves on down a series of tubes and reservoirs, such as the stomach, until it reaches the end of the colon – the anus. At each stage there are valves and peristaltic movements that ensure the food is always heading in the right direction. Problems with any valve or part of the system can disrupt the whole process – this is usually signalled by constipation or diarrhea. While most of us occasionally suffer from these conditions, long periods or frequent attacks of constipation or diarrhea require medical attention.

LI 4

St 36

Magnets and constipation

The effectiveness of magnet therapy for constipation is difficult to evaluate, since most cases are relatively short-term and normality returns as soon as the body regulates itself, with or without external assistance. However, they can provide some relief. Place small magnets on the following acupuncture points: St 36 (on the outside of the leg just below the knee) and LI 4 (on the back of the hand on the "V" formed by the bones of the thumb meeting the bones of the first finger). Other positions that may help are: about 2 cm (1 in) either side of the umbilicus; on the top of each knee, on the center line of the leg at the front; and about 2 cm (1 in) above the top "fold" of the knee, on the center line.

Other therapies

Treatments which can successfully augment magnet therapy for constipation are:

- Acupuncture
- Dietary control
- Shiatsu

HABITUAL CONSTIPATION

Name: **Ronald**   Age: **74**

Symptoms

The main reason for Ronald's visit to the clinic was constipation. Retired, in general good health, with a comfortable lifestyle and a very healthy diet and exercise regime, Ronald had suffered from irregular bowel movements and hard stools for many years, although the problem had gradually worsened over the last year. His medical practitioner had prescribed laxatives and sent him for MRI scans, barium meal x-rays, and other tests, which had revealed no abnormalities.

Ronald was resigned to taking laxatives for life when a friend recommended a visit to a natural health clinic as a last resort. It transpired that Ronald's diet was a good mix of healthy foods involving fresh vegetables and fruit as well as meat and grain products. Liquid intake was low but his alcoholic consumption was reasonable.

In-depth discussion revealed that Ronald's problems had really started during his time in the army. His military duties often required him to be active for long periods without being able to empty the bowels. In combat situations, this was clearly a "normal" situation, and the allied adrenaline-fired mix of fear and excitement, together with irregular eating times and high-protein, compact foods, ensured long periods of disrupted bowel activity. It was agreed that learned behavior probably played a part in Ronald's constipation.

It seemed that his digestive system had learned how to restrict bowel movements and that the brain had learned that it was good to restrict them.

Treatment

Ronald was advised to drink a litre (two pints) of water every day, in addition to his usual fluid intake. For one week, he followed a low-fiber diet to rest the bowels and ensure they were not scoured by too much fiber. For the second week, a diet with more fruit in it than usual was recommended. In subsequent weeks, eating more fiber-containing foods for breakfast and walking for thirty minutes after breakfast was advised. During all this time, magnets were positioned as follows: **St 36** (on the outside of the leg just below the knee); **LI 4** (on the back of the hand on the "V" formed by the bones of the thumb meeting the bones of the first finger); about 2 cm (1 in) **either side of the umbilicus**; **above each knee**, on the center line of the leg at the front, about 2 cm (1 in) above the top "fold" of the knee, on the center line (see illustration on page 79).

After the first week, some improvement was gained and slowly, over the next few months, Ronald's constipation gradually improved.

Insomnia

Insomnia is the inability to fall asleep or to remain asleep for an acceptable length of time; it is not the same as being prevented from sleeping by pain or external factors. Although certain illnesses can bring on insomnia, anxiety and stress are the usual causes. They force the brain to be overactive at a time when the body needs rest and sleep. When this situation occurs for prolonged periods our brains can learn that sleep is "wrong" and should be avoided.

Other sleep disorders

Sleep apnea is not insomnia, although some of the symptoms are similar. Nor is it just snoring: it is a dangerous condition where the patient stops breathing while they are sleeping. The body reacts to this by forcing the sufferer into near wakefulness, and this can happen as often as seven hundred times a night. If the body fails to react quickly enough when it occurs, then serious harm or even death can result. In any case, the continual spells of "holding the breath" put an enormous strain on the heart. A patient with sleep apnea also finds it difficult to stay awake and concentrate during the day.

COPD, or chronic obstructive pulmonary disease, will also cause insomnia-type symptoms. As with sleep apnea, the ability of the patient to breathe normally should be thoroughly investigated before a diagnosis of insomnia is made.

Narcolepsy is another, fortunately very rare, disease with some insomnia-type symptoms. It should be eliminated from the picture before treatment. Narcolepsy is defined as sleep at inappropriate times, which is usually accompanied by, but at different times, a condition known as cataplexy, when the patient stays awake but very suddenly is temporarily paralyzed. This can last from a few seconds up to several minutes.

Warning

Before treating for insomnia, check with your medical practitioner that your symptoms are not caused by another condition.

Treating insomnia

The first step is to determine whether the condition is due to a temporary worry, a deep-seated anxiety or a learned pattern of behavior that is no longer appropriate.

Using magnets on the following selected points on wrists and ankles may help:

K 6 Just under the ankle bone on the inside of the foot.

Sp 6 About 8 cm or 3 in above the ankle bone and just to the back of the shin bone.

B 62 Just below the ankle bone on the outside of the foot.

LI 4 On the back of the hand at the "V" formed by the bone of the thumb meeting that of the first finger.

H 7 On the inside of the wrist on the crease towards the small finger, just inside the bone that can be felt there.

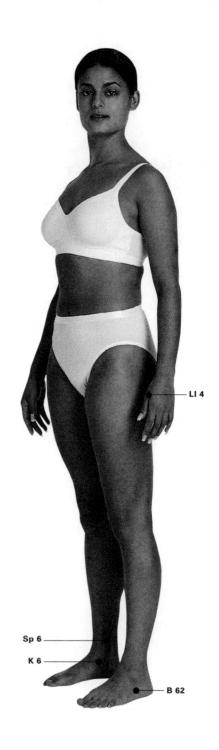

LI 4

Sp 6

K 6

B 62

Other therapies

Treatments which can successfully augment magnet therapy for insomnia are:

- Hypnotism
- Yoga
- Reflexology
- Aromatherapy

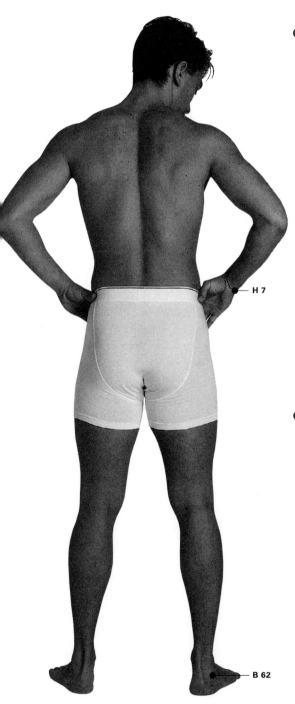

● ● ● ● ● ● ● ●

General advice for insomniacs

- Avoid coffee and other stimulants which contain caffeine after lunchtime.
- Avoid heavy meals after 6 pm.
- Check that your bed and pillows are comfortable; too soft a bed and too many thick pillows can result in a lack of sleep.
- Try to keep regular waking and sleeping hours.
- Make sure the temperature in your room does not fluctuate too much during the night.
- Only go to bed to sleep when you are tired and ready to sleep.
- If you wake up and cannot get back to sleep, do not toss and turn, waiting to fall asleep. Get up and keep yourself occupied with low-level physical activities, such as reading, watching television or doing crosswords, until you feel sleepy again.

● ● ● ● ● ● ● ●

Sleeping on magnets

Some people advocate placing magnets under the pillow at night. Although this may work for some, it is the action and the expectation of positive results that may be effective rather than anything that the magnets do in this case.

DEPRESSION AND LISTLESSNESS

Name: **Fiona**   Age: **52**

Symptoms

Fiona came to the clinic because she felt constantly tired, depressed and listless, and was very aware of her own irritability and short temper. Discussion revealed that she was post-menopausal and that although she had considerable emotional stress and feelings of guilt, she was happy with her life. However, she was afraid that her bad temper and listlessness would adversely affect her relationships with those she loved. Her medical practitioner had prescribed standard anti-depressive medication, but this was not the type of treatment she wished to take.

Treatment

During two shiatsu treatments given a week apart, Fiona spoke about her emotional state. She felt that she had failed to meet her mother's expectations, and the resulting guilt was the root cause of her unnecessary pain and suffering.

It was suggested that Fiona keep a sleep diary, recording the times at which she went to bed, when she got up during the night, and in the mornings an impression of how much sleep she had had and how rested she felt. This revealed that she was sleeping very little and the sleep she did have was full of dreams and nightmares.

Fiona was advised to take up yoga, avoid stimulants, such as tea and coffee, in the evenings, and, whenever practical, sleep during the day for about an hour if she felt very tired and listless. Alternate shiatsu or aromatherapy treatments – one week shiatsu, the next week aromatherapy – were recommended.

Magnets were placed as follows: **K 6** just under the ankle bone on the inside of the foot; **Sp 6**, about 8 cm (3 in) above the ankle bone and just to the back of the shin bone; **B 62**, just below the ankle bone on the outside of the foot (see page 83); **LI 4**, on the back of the hand at the "V" formed by the bone of the thumb meeting that of the first finger; **at the base of the thumb** on the wrist crease on the inside of the wrist; **H 7**, on the inside of the wrist on the crease towards the small finger, just inside the bone (see page 83).

Fiona was also encouraged to talk about her mother's attitude to her with other members of her family. However, she found this stressful and it was postponed until she felt emotionally stronger.

Within three days of fixing the magnets, Fiona's sleep diary showed an improvement in the degree of rest she felt after sleeping. After a week, she no longer needed to sleep during the day, and was sleeping longer and with less vivid dreams. The underlying psychological causes of Fiona's insomnia would take long-term care, but the first objective of coping and reducing the adverse effects had been achieved.

STRESS-RELATED INSOMNIA

Name: **Ian** Age: **26**

Symptoms

Ian came to the clinic because his wife had encouraged him to. He complained of being unable to sleep, but did not want any treatment, and felt that he could solve the problem himself. He believed that stress at work was the cause of his insomnia. He worked long hours and drank coffee to aid his concentration. His diet was unbalanced, made up of snatched meals whenever possible. Once Ian was satisfied he was being treated by a qualified complementary practitioner, he expressed interest in magnet therapy, although he would not accept any form of massage.

Treatment

Magnets were used as described on page 84. Ian was asked to cut down the amount of coffee he drank after 5 pm and to record his sleep patterns. After three days, he reported that he had stopped drinking coffee from the afternoon onwards, had revised his schedules by starting work earlier in the morning, had allowed time for proper meals and had been on a two-mile walk every day. He was already sleeping better and feeling the benefits.

Five days later, Ian's wife telephoned, thanking the clinic for helping her husband get back to his normal self. The magnets had been removed after seven days but Ian was still sleeping better and regaining his former zest for life.

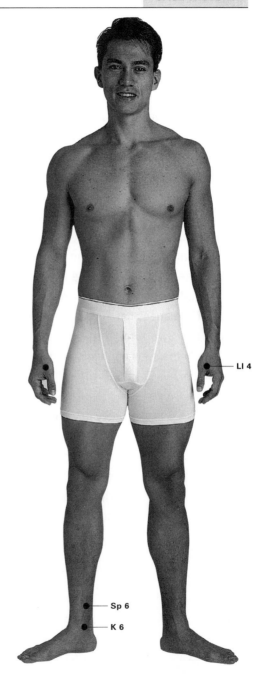

LI 4

Sp 6

K 6

Bronchitis

Bronchitis is the inflammation of the bronchial tubes that lead into the lungs. The lungs are rather like big sponges with two systems of tubes running through them. One tube system is a collection of blood vessels, and the other system is made up of tubes carrying oxygen-rich air in and waste gases out. The lungs transfer air gases into the blood, and unwanted gases out of the blood back out of the body. These air tubes start off relatively large and become progressively smaller as they feed into branches, rather as a tree has a large trunk, which becomes branches, each smaller in diameter than the trunk, and they then become even smaller twigs.

The bronchial tree is the system of tubes conducting air from the trachea (windpipe) to the lungs; the subdivisions are called the bronchi; the smaller tubes, the bronchioles. Bronchitis is caused by a virus that invades these air passages and causes a build-up of mucus. The patient has a cough, producing large amounts of mucus or sputum. Swabs of the mucus can be tested to indicate the presence of the virus and various medications are available to reduce the problem.

Symptoms of bronchitis

The fact that bronchitis is a relatively common condition does not mean that it can be neglected. Severe bronchitis can kill. The clogging of the air passages prevents oxygen reaching the blood and, therefore, reaching the muscles and brain where it is needed. The coughing spasms caused by the body's reflex action in trying to clear the tubes adds to the exhaustion and weakening of the patient. This weakening means that, even after the virus or bacteria has been fought and the mucus cleared from the tubes, the patient still needs restorative care. Recurring bronchitis indicates that the virus or bacteria has never fully cleared.

Warning

Smoking, air pollution and the lack of exercise and fresh air all encourage the bronchitis microbe to take root in the bronchial tubes.

Alleviating the symptoms

In the worst stages of the illness, a patient's breathing must be alleviated: medication, massage of the upper back, fresh air and, in many cases, the inhalation of moist vapor all help, as will anti-spasmodic cough syrups. Some patients find it easier to sleep sitting up. The traditional remedy of inhaling eucalyptus in boiling water may be beneficial, but should not be used for severe cases of bronchitis, as the water vapor will reduce the amount of available oxygen still further, and the patient's ability to take in oxygen may be reduced to dangerously low levels.

Treating with magnets

Magnets applied to the following places will help reduce the effects of the condition (see illustration on page 88): both sides of the chest, level with the bottom of the armpit, about 2–5 cm (1–2 in) in from the side of the body; on the points level with these but closer to the center of the body, either side of the breast bone; on the back in the center of each shoulder blade; close to, but either side of, the spine, about one-third of the way from the top of the shoulder blade; at the bottom of the shoulder blade, just off the spine and either side of it; Liv 3, on top of each foot, between the large toe and its neighbor, about 2 cm (1 in) up from the web (see page 89).

Other therapies
Treatments that can successfully augment magnet therapy for bronchitis are:
• Acupuncture
• Massage
• Shiatsu

RECURRING WINTER BRONCHITIS

Name: **Gerald**   Age: **48**

Symptoms

Gerald was in his late forties and suffered from recurring bouts of bronchitis about once a year, usually during the winter. Each year the attacks seemed to weaken him more and he took longer to recover from them. During the summer he was outdoors a great deal, gardening and walking, but the cold winter winds changed his lifestyle and he did very little by way of exercise or outdoor activity. His last attack of bronchitis had taken a couple of months to shake off, and another two months later, when he visited the clinic, he was still not fully fit.

Treatment

Discussion revealed that Gerald's winter diet was too full of dairy products for his relatively inactive lifestyle at this time of the year. The negative effect of the mucus build-up that his diet caused, combined with inactivity and little fresh air, were explained. Gerald agreed to change his diet and try to walk a mile a day, whatever the weather, but only on the understanding that he was not suffering from bronchitis at the time.

Gerald began taking garlic capsules as a once-a-day

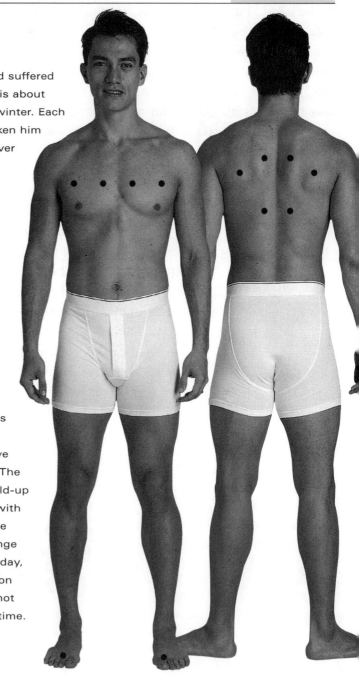

supplement, and root ginger was added as often as possible to the daily cooking. The merits of echinacea as a boost to the immune system, and cinnamon as a symptom-relieving agent, were also explained. Gerald was told that the benefits of these changes would take some time to be noticeable.

Magnets were applied on the following points: **both sides of the chest**, level with the bottom of the armpit, about 2–5 cm (1–2 in) in from the side of the body; on points level with these but **closer to the center of the body**, either side of the breast bone; on the back **in the center of each shoulder blade**; close to, but **either side of, the spine**, about one-third of the way from the top of the shoulder blade; at **the bottom of the shoulder blade**, just off the spine and either side of it; **Liv 3**, on top of the foot between the large toe and its neighbor, about 2 cm (1 in) up from the web.

Whenever the magnets became dislodged, they were replaced with adhesive surgical tape. Gerald understood the long-term nature of the treatment: the magnets were left in place for two weeks, removed for one week and replaced for two further weeks.

Gerald did suffer a bronchitis attack the following winter, but it was reduced in severity and duration. Magnets were applied during the attack and left in place until he was well. The changes in diet and exercise were maintained, and, in subsequent years, the attacks became less severe and debilitating.

CHILD'S BRONCHITIS

CASE HISTORY

Name: **Joshua**   Age: **9**

Symptoms

Joshua, suffering from a chesty, phlegmy cough, was brought to the clinic. His mother did not want him to be treated with antibiotics. She was giving him herbal preparations to relieve the symptoms. Physical examination at the clinic of the lung treatment points used in magnet therapy indicated that the slightest pressure on these points caused great pain. She was advised to take Joshua to their medical practitioner and have him checked for bronchitis.

Treatment

Magnets were supplied to Joshua's mother and she was shown where to position them (as described above and in the illustration opposite). She agreed to take Joshua to their medical practitioner for confirmation of the diagnosis and she then positioned the magnets. A week later, she called to say that Joshua's bronchitis had eased within forty-eight hours of the magnets being applied, and that there had been a continual gradual improvement since then.

Muscle strain

Most muscles are made up of bundles of stretchy fibers that can shorten by up to one-third when they contract. Muscle strains occur when the muscles are required to contract against a load that is too great for them, or asked to do too many contractions within a short period of time.

There are more than three hundred muscles in the human body, which make up forty per cent of healthy body weight. Some muscles, such as the heart, work without conscious brain commands. Others exist to make joints move and to hold body parts in certain positions. These do require conscious brain commands.

Muscles can only contract and relax (they can only pull and do not push), so each muscle has a corresponding partner to move the body part back to its original position. For example, one muscle moves the arm up, while another moves it down. These two muscles are always in a degree of tension as they interact with each other to hold a limb in a particular position.

Detecting muscle strain

Muscle strains are not the same as muscle tears, but telling the difference between them is not always that easy. The situation can be complicated by the presence of a strained joint or ligament; sometimes it is not the muscle that is strained but the connective tissue joining the muscle to the bone or joint. Torn muscles bleed internally, and this must be stopped before applying magnets or heat, or massaging. Strained muscles, on the other hand, need magnets, heat and massage.

A completely torn muscle will produce great pain and loss of movement, while a strained muscle will cause some pain and discomfort but mobility will be possible, if uncomfortable. A torn muscle requires

---

Warning

Inflammation is the body's response to attack; the symptoms are swelling, pain and, often, heat. If inflammation is evident and persistent, then consult your medical practitioner as it may be due to infection rather than to a strain.

---

urgent medical treatment as surgery may be needed, but a cold compress is a good first-aid treatment if medical help is not immediately available. A strained muscle, on the other hand, can be treated with hot, or alternate hot and cold, poultices. Strains often become apparent some time after the activity stops, while a torn muscle is usually apparent immediately.

Treatment

Treating a muscle strain with magnets is best done with either a magnetic bandage wrapped around the injured part of the limb or, if the strained muscle is on the torso, with small magnets positioned around the area of pain, with one or two additional ones at the center of this area.

Test the extent of the damage by gentle pressure and by determining which movements cause pain. If you need to use extra tape to hold the magnets in place, or if you are using a magnetic bandage, do not be tempted to over-tighten them: support is good, restricting the blood flow is not. Keeping warm, hot baths, massage, shiatsu, aromatherapy, rest and avoiding overworking the injured part are all advisable. Taking painkillers and anti-inflammatory medications is sometimes necessary but beware of thinking that masking the pain with medication is a sign that the damaged part can be overused again.

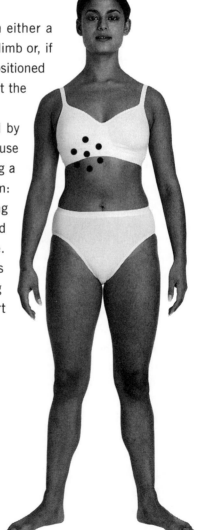

Other therapies

Treatments which can successfully augment magnet therapy for muscle strain are:

- Massage
- Physiotherapy
- Rest
- Aromatherapy

LEG STRAIN

Name: **Daniel**   Age: **20**

Symptoms

Daniel called in at the clinic nursing a painful leg. Although a football enthusiast who played amateur matches on Sunday mornings, trained twice a week for two hours and went dancing on Saturday nights, Daniel otherwise led a fairly sedentary life. He could not remember any particular knock or moment that might have caused an injury. It was normal for him to feel stiff and bruised after playing football, and so he had not noticed this particular discomfort until he tried to train again more than two days or so after the last match. He then felt pain in the right thigh, particularly on the outside, which prevented him from training, so he rested until the Thursday night and tried to train again. The pain was still there and he contacted the clinic the next morning.

Treatment

A physical examination and an assessment of Daniel's mobility revealed that the problem was a strain to the muscles and nothing more serious. A magnetic bandage was wrapped around the thigh, and small magnets were stuck to the **top of the foot**, about 2 cm (1 in) above the web between the large toe and its neighbor, and to the extreme outside of the hip, at the widest point across the hips. These were placed on the injured side of the body only. He was advised that walking would encourage blood flow to the site of the injury and reduce muscle wastage.

Daniel missed the match on the following Sunday but he was able to train on the Tuesday, with the magnetic bandage temporarily removed and replaced with support strapping. After the post-training shower, he put the magnets and bandage back on in the positions he had been advised.

The next day, Daniel experienced some stiffness, but followed the advice about walking which helped matters. The same routine was repeated for his next training session and he was able to play the following Sunday match, with the thigh strapped up. After wearing the magnets and bandage in the same way for another week, Daniel was fully recovered.

STRAIN

Name: **Laura**   Age: **36**

Symptoms

Laura, a very fit aerobics teacher, was experiencing pain and discomfort in her left shoulder. Her diet was strictly vegetarian and she did not smoke, drink alcohol or eat sugary foods. She had a somewhat dogmatic outlook to her lifestyle. It was, therefore, no surprise that Laura's pain and the restrictions it put on her physical movement caused her a disproportionate amount of mental anguish. She really did seem to believe that she should never be ill or suffer injury because she was living the "right" way. Apart from a need for counselling over this attitude to herself and others, the first priority was to reduce the pain and discomfort, and so repair her damaged self-esteem.

Treatment

Aromatherapy massage was used to relax the physical tension created by Laura's response to the problem. Between each session, small magnets were adhered to **the "point" of her left shoulder**. Four other magnets were also placed down the edge of her left shoulder blade, **between the spine and the shoulder blade**.

Laura reported reduced discomfort within a day and she resumed her teaching. After a week she was back to full mobility, with only slight discomfort. She continued to use the magnets for a further ten days, and then wore the magnets only at night for a further two weeks. By this time Laura was fully recovered.

Stress

Stress can be physical or emotional, but mostly we consider it to be a mental problem with physical side effects. The best definition of stress is the effect of high demands combined with low levels of control over a particular situation. When people who matter to us expect things we cannot achieve, or when unreasonable demands are made of us, we become stressed. But it is not the demands themselves or the expectations that create the stress, it is our failure or inability to control the situation.

Chronic stress has a cumulative effect. The daily problems at work may not increase and the difficulties of living on a low income do not change overnight, but a person may suddenly find themselves no longer able to cope with the situation. It is like a jug being filled with water. Everything is fine until the top of the jug is reached and then suddenly the water overflows.

Positive stress

A moderate degree of stress is generally seen to be desirable in most people, as it helps to motivate and generate creativity. Reversely, too much stress can overload our capacity to cope with situations and it can become dangerous, particularly if the stress impinges on our safety or that of others.

Warning

Symptoms of stress can also be indicative of other physical disorders and should be checked by your medical practitioner. For example, one symptom of liver dysfunction is anger. Diabetes may also produce similar symptoms, so blood sugar levels should be checked by a medical practitioner.

The effects of stress

The physical results of stress may include muscular stiffness, digestive problems, raised blood pressure, insomnia, perpetual tiredness, reduced eyesight, reduced libido, hair loss and skin complaints. Emotional results of stress may include irritability, bad temper, mood swings, irrationality, lack of consideration for others and the misjudgement of others' motives and feelings.

Rebuilding self-esteem

Although the mental and physical effects of stress are very variable, relaxation and the rebuilding of damaged self-esteem are essential. A period of calm and "time out" is usually beneficial. This may be only half an hour a day for a mother of young children, but it helps to have some time that is yours alone, where the focus is on you, your feelings and your needs.

Treating with magnets

Magnets can help with the physical effects of stress by reducing muscular tension. Magnets can also help in more subtle ways, reducing the emotional effects of raised stress levels. To help reduce stress caused by external influences, such as pressure at work or financial difficulty, position four magnets on the back, just below the bottom of the shoulder blade and either side of the spine, about 2 cm (1 in) and 5 cm (2 in) in from the center line of the spine. To help with internal stress resulting from the demands we place on ourselves, stick the magnets at the top of the shoulder blades just below the top line of the shoulder and just above the top ridge of the shoulder blade.

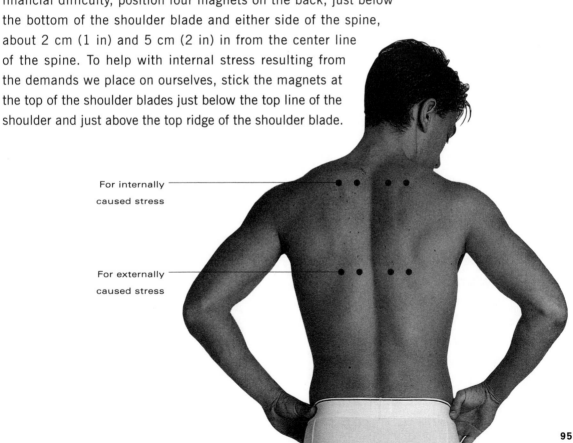

For internally caused stress

For externally caused stress

WORK-RELATED STRESS

Name: **Anthony**   Age: **40**

Symptoms

Anthony came to the clinic because he felt that his powers of concentration were deteriorating. He revealed that he worked long hours at a demanding sales job and relied on commission to earn what he termed a "reasonable" wage. He argued with his wife, suffered from headaches and was perpetually tired. These revelations helped Anthony see that all these things were connected. His work was driven by the need to be better than other employees and to be better than he was himself the previous year. Although this motivational style may gain an employer short-term results, it has a destructive effect on employees as they realize that they have no actual control over the demands of work. This creates stress.

Other therapies

Treatments which can successfully augment magnet therapy for stress are:

- Relaxation techniques
- Shiatsu
- Aromatherapy
- Massage
- Reflexology

Treatment

Anthony regarded physical therapies as acceptable forms of treatment, but did not feel comfortable with relaxation techniques, as suggested by his wife. Massage and shiatsu were therefore used. The muscular tensions associated with stress and the "body armor" we generate to hold in our inner tensions soon became apparent in Anthony. The pain and discomfort that he felt during these treatments were enough to convince him that he was undergoing a "real" treatment regime that would bring about physical change.

Magnets were used between the massage treatments. Small magnets were placed in two columns, about 2 cm (1 in) apart **either side of the spine**, starting about 2 cm (1 in) above the top of the shoulder blade and extending to about 5 cm (2 in) below the bottom of the shoulder blade (see illustration right).

The combination of talking, massage, shiatsu and magnets had an immediate effect on Anthony. He stopped arguing with his wife, started to sleep better and lost the feeling of tiredness within three days. After a month, Anthony reported that he no longer experienced any of the other symptoms. He stopped using the magnets, but he and his wife joined a gym where they not only had weekly, unwinding workouts but also monthly shiatsu sessions.

FINANCIAL STRESS

Name: **Emily**   Age: **25**

Symptoms

Emily, an unemployed single mother, reported all sorts of aches and pains that had no obvious physical cause. Her medical practitioner recommended anti-depressants and a visit to the local depression treatment clinic, but this had a three-month waiting list. Discussion showed that Emily's financial situation was causing her great stress. She existed on state benefits, had no savings and felt insecure about all aspects of her life. Her self-esteem was very low.

Treatment

Emily could not afford to join a gym, or undergo physical treatments that would have been beneficial, but she did have a friend with children in a similar position. They set up a system to give each other 'time out'. This involved Emily looking after both sets of children one morning a week while her friend used this time just for herself, and not doing housework or shopping unless she actually wanted to. The following morning they swapped roles.

Magnets were also used in two columns, about 2 cm (1 in) apart **either side of the spine**, starting about 2 cm (1 in) above the top of the shoulder blade and extending to about 5 cm (2 in) below the bottom of the shoulder blade. They were kept in place for ten days, removed for three days and then put back on for a further ten days.

Emily's financial problems did not go away but she did find it easier to cope with them. She became more relaxed with her children and started to enjoy life.

Nausea

Nausea is the feeling that you are about to be sick, and vomiting is the reflex action of ejecting the contents of the stomach out through the mouth. Nausea may persist without actual vomiting and it can continue after vomiting has occurred.

Causes of nausea

Vomiting is controlled by the brain, and the brain may be acting on a signal from the stomach or the inner ear. The latter triggers both travel sickness and nausea caused by vertigo. The signals from the stomach are usually triggered by eating or drinking irritants. A strong emotional reaction to something may cause the brain to trigger the reflex action, such as the thought of eating something that you regard as really revolting. What the stomach regards as an irritant can be an excess of something it can usually cope with, such as alcohol, or it may be an unwanted agent, such as a virus or bacteria.

Pregnancy can often cause nausea and vomiting. Although it is commonly known as "morning sickness," nausea during pregnancy is not confined to the mornings. Some women do not suffer from it at all, while an unfortunate few experience it for the whole of their pregnancy. Anesthetics are another possible cause of nausea, and "post-operative nausea" may slow down a patient's recovery from an operation.

Many people have successfully used magnets to prevent travel sickness. Where treatment has been unsuccessful, it appears that the magnets have not been maintained in the correct position; a loose magnetic band moving about the wrist will have no effect on the relevant acupuncture points.

Warning

The persistent feeling of nausea or sickness should be checked by a medical practitioner. Prolonged sickness can cause dehydration. It is important to drink water if the vomiting has lasted for any length of time. If you cannot keep water down for more than twenty-four hours, contact your doctor immediately.

Increasing the pressure

If your magnets are in place and a wave of nausea starts to sweep over you, try pressing the magnets. This introduces an acupressure element to help cope with the increase in the problem.

Preventing nausea

Avoiding foods that you know irritate your stomach is an obvious way of preventing nausea in the first place. If this is impossible, try taking slippery elm (the bark of the red elm, available from health food stores), to prevent the irritants coming into contact with the stomach wall. There are other medications available without prescription containing inert materials that do the same job.

Treating with magnets

To stop the reflex action of vomiting, position magnets on P 6 (on the center line on the inside of the forearm, about three fingers' width up from the wrist crease, between the two tendons); and on the wrist crease itself, on the center line inside the forearm.

   To reduce the feeling of nausea, position magnets on the wrist crease itself, on the center line inside the forearm; on the front of the trunk of the body, either side of the center line, about 2 cm (1 in) from that center line, one-third of the distance down from the nipples to the umbilicus; on the front center line of the body, halfway between the umbilicus and the nipples; about 2 cm (1 in) above the previously positioned magnet.

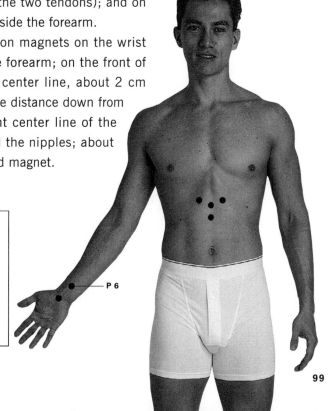

Other therapies

Treatments which can successfully augment magnet therapy for nausea are:

- Acupuncture
- Shiatsu

P 6

MORNING SICKNESS

Name: **Gabrielle**   Age: **23**

Symptoms

Gabrielle was two months pregnant when she called at the clinic. Morning sickness was dominating her life; she felt constantly sick and ill, was unable to work and was not enjoying her pregnancy at all. After following advice to consult her medical practitioner and visit the antenatal clinic, it was established that Gabrielle was perfectly healthy and that hormonal changes were probably the cause of her nausea.

Treatment

Magnets were stuck to the insides of Gabrielle's wrists on **P 6** (on the center line on the inside of the forearm, about three fingers' width up from the wrist crease, between the two tendons); and **on the wrist crease itself**, on the center line inside the forearm (see illustration). The feeling of nausea did not completely disappear but it was reduced to a tolerable level. After another month, Gabrielle's body seemed to have passed through this particular stage of her pregnancy and the feeling of nausea stopped altogether.

POST-OPERATIVE NAUSEA

Name: **Brian**   Age: **79**

Symptoms and treatment

Brian, who was recovering after a hospital operation, was troubled by nausea. Magnets were placed on the insides of his wrists, as described above, and within two days, his nausea had completely disappeared.

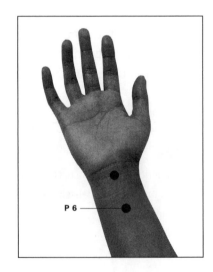

P 6

DIET-RELATED NAUSEA

Name: **Adam**   Age: **21**

Symptoms

Adam came to the clinic complaining of always feeling sick. He had consulted his medical practitioner who had carried out various tests but had not offered any remedial treatment. Discussion revealed that Adam had a chaotic eating pattern, and his meals were usually junk food, taken at snatched moments, often standing up or while driving. Adam was highly strung, a talented musician who lived only for his music. Mentally, he almost disregarded his physical body, except that the nausea was affecting his concentration and consequently his work.

Treatment

Adam agreed to wear magnets on his wrists, as described left, and on the following points: on the **front of the trunk of the body**, either side of the center line, about 2 cm (1 in) from that center line, one-third of the distance down from the nipples to the umbilicus; on the front center line of the body, **halfway between the navel and the nipples**; and about **2 cm (1 in) above this**. He also agreed to take up yoga as a way of relaxing his body. He had a couple of shiatsu sessions, although his travelling and work schedules prevented regular treatment. Adam replaced the magnets after showering and he kept them in place for at least seven days, as directed. After this time, Adam reported that the nausea had reduced and that he was making an effort to improve his eating habits and allow time for food to digest before any stressful activities. The magnets were used on a cycle of seven days on and five days off for a further three weeks. A while later he called at the clinic to say that he no longer had the symptoms.

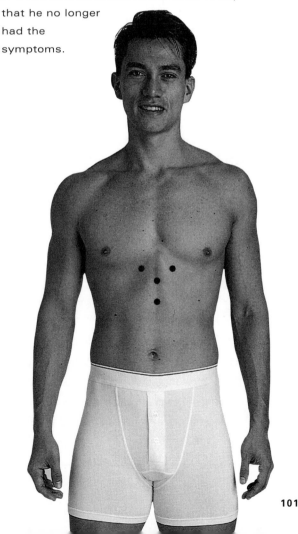

Additional magnet information

Using magnets with other treatments

To restrict the speed of recovery by using only one treatment at a time, usually on the pretext of ensuring you know what is working, can be unfair to a patient. The primary object of healthcare is to promote as rapid and as safe a recovery as possible. But an important secondary objective is to ensure that the quality and enjoyability of life are maximized during treatment. In some specific instances, particularly during chemotherapy treatment for cancer, the treatment may reduce the quality of life on a temporary basis in order to achieve the primary objective.

Combining therapies to improve the speed of recovery makes a great deal of sense. Relatively low-costing and self-administered natural treatments, combined with modern medication and intervention techniques, can provide a quicker and better improvement than the sum of the individual treatments would suggest. In all medical and health matters, however, nothing is certain. Each person is so individual, their chemical metabolism and psychological reactions so variable, that broad claims of any certainty cannot be made.

The holistic approach

In much modern conventional medicine, the removal of a particular set of named symptoms is seen as a "cure." The fact that the same patient may have another set of symptoms which remain uncured, does not affect the claim. Practitioners of holistic and natural medicine, on the other hand, are usually reluctant to use the term "cure" because they do not see the removal of one set of symptoms as signifying the patient is now in perfect good health. The underlying causes of poor health may still exist, and so the same set of symptoms, or a different manifestation of the cause disguised as a new set of symptoms, may appear at any time. This is not a new illness, just the old one re-formed.

Working with other treatments

As can be seen from the real case histories included in this book magnet therapy can be used with other forms of treatment. Using magnets between, for example, shiatsu,

---

Warning

Do not use magnets if you are fitted with a pacemaker or other electromechanical device. Do not store magnets close to homeopathic remedies. (However, magnet therapy and homeopathic treatments can be used as part of a combined treatment.)

---

massage, aromatherapy or reflexology treatments, has the beneficial effect of enhancing the therapeutic value of all the other treatments involved. Flower remedies, which are wonderful for treating the emotional and mental effects of poor health, combined with magnet therapy, which treats the direct physical problems, can provide a balanced holistic treatment. Taking herbal medicines while wearing magnets will enhance the effect of both. Chemical drug medications should not normally be adversely affected by the wearing of small magnets at selected points.

Using painkillers as a coping strategy, while allowing magnets and other treatments time to work, is sensible and safe, provided that the recommended dosage is followed, that you do not use painkillers you are allergic to, or for prolonged periods.

Electromagnetic devices

Electromagnetic devices, which provide intermittent pulses or waves of magnetic force, are becoming ever more popular and sophisticated. Increased waves of magnetic induction can assist body tissue to absorb the required material from such things as herbal tonics, showing that the combined effect of various therapies used simultaneously can be greater than the effect of an individual therapy.

The experienced, technically proficient manufacturers do take great care to ensure that the electromagnetic devices they sell can have only beneficial effects. The potential for a powerful electromagnetic device to harm is very great, and caution should be exercised when you are around, or in contact with, these pieces of equipment. The manufacturers of powerful industrial transmitters do not allow staff to work on them while they are active for very good reasons.

Using caution

There are very few things with the power to heal that do not have the power to cause harm as well. The fact that something can effect changes indicates that it also has the ability to make undesired or inappropriate changes, which could be damaging.

Treating broken bones

Combining magnet therapy with mechanical intervention and painkilling medications, as a short-term coping strategy for the treatment of broken bones, will speed up the mending process. If a broken limb is in rigid plaster, small magnets can be placed above and below the plastered area. If the injury is strapped or bound with support bandaging, the magnets can be placed within this. Remember to remove the magnets if x-rays are to be taken!

By ensuring you eat a balanced diet, use herbal remedies and food supplements, the whole healing process should be speeded up and the mended bones should be stronger.

Vitamin C is needed throughout life for the repair of any body tissue. It is needed in increased amounts when we are ill or suffering from injury. The repair of broken bones requires calcium and other micronutrients. These should be present in large enough quantities in any healthy diet, but during the repair and rejuvenation process, any shortcoming in your diet will delay or weaken the repair work.

Magnets can be used to help improve blood flow and the delivery of repair materials to the site of the damage. Your diet must provide these repair materials, one of which is calcium. This is available to the body in a variety of foods, not just milk; the stems of green vegetables, for example, are rich in calcium. There are many good nutritional guides and as many businesses selling food supplements. If you are in any doubt about how good your diet is and whether you should take food supplements, ask your medical practitioner or seek out a qualified nutritionist.

Weight loss during the aftermath of a trauma injury is another condition that must be looked into carefully; a loss of more than ten per cent of body weight in these circumstances can be clinically significant. Research has shown that under-nutrition affects mood and causes depression which, in turn, affects appetite, resulting in a vicious circle.

Treating menstrual pains

Magnet therapy for the relief of menstrual pains can be enhanced by the use of tissue salts, correctly named "biochemic tissue salts," which are homeopathic-type medications. Mag Phos (*Magnesia phosphorica*) will help to reduce the cramp-like pains.

Rheumatism and arthritis

Some experts advocate certain diets to help reduce the painful effects of rheumatism and arthritis. They believe that all forms of rheumatic pain are caused by a disturbance of the acid-alkaline balance in the body, and that this disturbance arises from faults in nutrition. They claim that a diet emphasizing alkaline-forming foods reduces the problem. Such a diet can be used in conjunction with magnets placed on the painful site. The changes in diet will have a slow and long-term effect, while the use of magnets may be a good short-term coping strategy while the dietary changes take full effect.

Treating stress

The treatment of stress by a combination of magnets and flower remedies is highly recommended. By using magnets, on the back as described on pages 94–97, and by taking the flower remedy Olive, for physical and mental renewal, together with another flower remedy that is specific to the nature of the patient, will bring great benefit.

Effects of magnets on plant growth

Over the years, experiments have taken place to establish the effects of magnets on other living organisms, such as plants. The ability of magnetic fields to influence growth rates gives an indication of their power to improve the flows of nutrients and to enhance organic energy, that is, the energy grown within an organism.

Experimenting with magnets

One simple "kitchen-table" experiment that you can conduct yourself is to part-fill three small plant pots all to the same level with compost, and then sow a few mustard seeds in each pot. Mark each pot with a number or letter. Place a magnet under the first pot with the north-seeking pole touching the base of the pot. Under the second pot, place an identical magnet but with the south-seeking pole touching the pot. The magnets in children's experiment kits are ideal for this. Do not place a magnet under the third pot. Water each pot with the same amount of water at the same times, always drawing the water from the same supply. Keep a record of the time it takes for the first growth to appear and then measure the growth each day for about a week.

You will almost certainly see a difference in the growth in the three pots. The pot with the north-seeking pole of the magnet touching will show the healthiest growth; the pot with no magnet underneath will show the next best growth; and the pot with the south-seeking pole will contain the least healthy-looking seedlings. The experiment shows that magnets do affect growth rates, and that the polarity of the magnet affects growth rates in different ways.

Magnetized water

As the name suggests, magnetized water is water that has been subjected to magnetic influence. However, it does not become magnetic itself in the way that an iron bar will become a magnet if subjected to magnetic forces.

Why drink magnetized water?

Drinking magnetized water for as long as an ailment lasts is recommended by many who have worked with magnets and healing. Some experimentation over the amount consumed and the time the water is exposed to the magnets may be needed to determine what is most beneficial to each individual patient. The strength of the magnets used will also be influential in this situation. Many exponents of magnet therapy recommend making separate quantities of water magnetized by each pole and mixing these in equal quantities before drinking. They suggest that an adult should drink 60 ml (2 fl oz) before breakfast and the same amount again after lunch and the evening meal. Plants watered with magnetized water may also have a better growth rate than otherwise.

How to magnetize water

Water can be subjected to magnetic influence by suspending a magnet over an empty jar and then slowly pouring water over the magnet into the jar. Alternatively, you can place a magnet in a jar of water and leave it there for a minimum of eight hours. The drawback of this method is that the magnet must be sterile and not left in the water long enough for it to rust as this could dangerously contaminate the liquid. A third way is to place a flat-bottomed jar, filled with water, on a magnet and leave it there for a minimum of eight hours before drinking. It has been suggested that water magnetized with the north pole against the base of a jar will have a different effect from water treated with the south pole against the base of the jar, although this is yet to be proved.

Glossary

acupuncture traditional Chinese treatment of disorders using the insertion of needle tips into the skin at specific points along the meridians.

acute describes a disease of rapid onset, severe symptoms and brief duration (compare with "chronic").

atom a small particle, once thought to be the smallest possible unit of anything and indivisible, but now known to comprise a central core and rotating electrons.

cartilage dense connective tissue that is very strong. There are several kinds of specialist cartilage in the body. The "connective" function is most important. When damaged, it does not repair itself easily.

chiropractic a system of treating body disorders by manipulation of the spine.

chronic describes a disease of long duration involving slow changes, often gradual onset (compare with "acute").

electromagnetic induction movement of a magnet around a copper wire induces an electric current in the wire. This is usually done by rotating a magnet inside a coil of wire to produce electrical current within the coil. The movement (kinetic) energy of the magnet is transformed into electrical energy within the wire coil.

element one of the fundamental, or irreducible components or substances, making up a whole.

enzyme a protein that, in small amounts, acts as a catalyst; it speeds up or facilitates a biological process in the body without being used up itself in the reaction. There are many enzymes which are vital for the body to function, such as those used in the digestive process.

free radical an oxygen-derived molecule that is unstable, which means it tries to latch on to other molecules to reach stability, and in the process can damage the molecule on to which it latches. Free radicals are used by the body as part of the defense system, but they also contribute to the ageing process and damage tissue. It is widely believed that pollution and modern urban lifestyles are causing increased exposure to free radicals.

gauss a unit used to measure the relative strength of magnets. For example, an 800-gauss magnet is four times as strong as a 200-gauss magnet. An alternative measure is the tesla. One tesla equals 10,000 gauss.

haemoglobin the molecule that causes the red blood cells to be red, and is the medium that allows oxygen to be transported within the body.

hormone a chemical messenger that carries information and signals around the body.

ion (ionic exchange) an electrically charged atom or group of atoms. Ionic exchange is the mechanism which allows these electrically charged particles to pass from a solution on to an insoluble solid.

ligament band or sheet of tough connective tissue that connects bones or cartilage, supports muscles, or restricts movement at joints.

meridian a pathway of energy within the body used in traditional Chinese medicine. Energy flows around the body in a continuous cycle. Most "maps" of meridians do not show them linked together for simplicity, although they do link up to form a continuous single path that conducts energy all around the body.

moxibustion the traditional Chinese process of applying heat to acupuncture points in order to gain therapeutic effects.

osteopathy a system of healing based on the manipulation of bones, muscles and joints.

physiology the science of the functioning of living organisms; how we look at the way the physical body works.

protein an organic compound that is an essential constituent of all living organisms, made up of amino acids. There are many kinds of proteins used in the body, each fulfilling some specialized task (see enzyme). Some proteins form the structural material of muscles. The body makes the proteins it requires by breaking down the proteins in our food into amino acids, and then re-combining selected amino acids into the particular proteins that the body needs at that time.

tendon inelastic tissue that attaches muscles to bones or some other part.

tissue a collection of various cells that group together to make up a specialized part of the body (such as muscle), in order to form a particular function (such as movement). Aggregations of tissue make up the organs (such as the heart). Connective tissue supports organs and fills the spaces between them, and forms tendons and ligaments.

vertebra one of thirty-three bones that make up the spine (backbone). Each vertebra has a hole in it, allowing the spinal cord to pass up the spine to the brain. The vertebra are separated by discs of cartilage that prevent them rubbing against each other.

Further reading

Healing with Magnets, Gary Null. London: Robinson Publishing, 1998.

Magnetic Cure for Common Diseases, Dr H.L. Bansal and Dr R.S. Bansal. Delhi: Orient Paperbacks, 1983.

Magnet Therapy, Ron Lawrence, Paul Rosch and Judith Plowden. Rocklin, California: Prima Publishing, 1998.

Magnet Therapy, Holger Hannemann. New York: Sterling Publishing, 1990.

Index

Acknowledgements

Author's Acknowledgements

The author would like to thank the following
organizations that have supplied information
that have greatly assisted in the writing of this
book: Digital Health Research Ltd; Magnetic
Applications Ltd; Magnetic Therapy Ltd;
Snowdon Healthcare Ltd; Dulwich Health.

Eddison•Sadd Editions

Eddison Sadd Editions would like to thank
Richard Whitehead and Magnetic Therapy Ltd
for providing the products shown on page 13.

Commissioning Editor Liz Wheeler
Editors Nicola Hodgson and Helen Ridge
Proofreader Michele Turney
Indexer Helen Smith
Art Director Elaine Partington
Senior Art Editor Hayley Cove
Art Editor Rachel Kirkland
Production Karyn Claridge and Charles James

Photographs on page 13 by Stephen Marwood
Models Michael Cooper and Melody
Woodhead

Resources

Suppliers of magnetic devices and equipment

Magnetsheal.com
239 Acoma Street 106
Denver
Colorado 80223
Tel: 303 722 1434
Info@magnetsheal.com
www.magnetsheal.com

Nikken Inc.
10866 Wilshire Boulevard
Suite 250
Los Angeles
California 90024
Tel: 310 446 4300

Enviro-Tech Products
17171 SE 29th Street
Choctaw
Oklahoma 73020
Tel: 405 390 2968

Bioflex Medical Magnets Inc.
3370 NE Fifth Avenue
Oakland Park
Florida 33334
Tel: 954 565 8500
Info@bioflexmagnets.com

Where to find a practitioner

Thomas Szulc Md.
720 Old Cantry Road
Plainview
NY 11803
Tel: 516 931 1133

Advanced Magnetic Research Institute
195 Stock Street
Hanover
PA 17331
Tel: 717 632 0300
www.amripa.com

AMRITUCSON.com

For your free set of magnets

So you can experience magnet therapy, we are providing you with five small-but-powerful magnets that can be applied anywhere on your body, from toes, fingers, ankles and elbows to knees, hips, tailbone and collarbone.

These are spot magnets like those widely available at health and fitness stores and used in the healing diagrams found in this book. Each spot magnet includes an adhesive backing that holds the magnet securely and comfortably in place.

For these free magnets, simply send us the receipt from the purchase of this book along with your name and address to:

Free Magnet Offer
Ulysses Press
P.O. Box 3440
Berkeley, CA 94703

(Additional sets of five healing spot magnets are available for $5)